TRAINING YOUR OWN SERVICE DOG
THE COMPLETE GUIDE SERIES
PUBLIC ACCESS SKILLS WORKBOOK

MEGAN BROOKS

COPYRIGHT © 2022 BY MEGAN BROOKS
ALL RIGHT RESERVED.

ALL RIGHTS RESERVED. ISBN: 9798428737240
IMPRINT: HELPING PAWS PUBLISHING CO.

NO PART OF THIS PUBLICATION MAY BE REPRODUCED, DISTRIBUTED, OR TRANSMITTED IN ANY FORM OR BY ANY MEANS FOR PROFIT, INCLUDING PHOTOCOPYING, RECORDING, OR OTHER ELECTRONIC OR MECHANICAL METHODS, OR BY ANY INFORMATION STORAGE AND RETRIEVAL SYSTEM WITHOUT THE PRIOR WRITTEN PERMISSION OF THE PUBLISHER, EXCEPT IN THE CASE OF VERY BRIEF QUOTATIONS EMBODIED IN CRITICAL REVIEWS AND CERTAIN OTHER NONCOMMERCIAL USES PERMITTED BY COPYRIGHT LAW.

THIS BOOK WAS PUBLISHED THANKS TO FREE SUPPORT AND TRAINING FROM:
TCKPUBLISHING.COM

Download the worksheets FREE!
https://drive.google.com/drive/folders/1ruuEKaNjoH2GflAtE2dr8V1I-53Ef6Zt?usp=sharing

CONTENTS

MegaLearn System 4 Phases..8

Lesson Training Sequence...9

Public Access Prerequisites...10

Chapter 1: What Qualifies My Dog as a Service Dog?

    Service Dog-in-Training vs. Full-fledged Service Dog..11

    So, When does an SDiT become a service dog?..14

    State Laws..15

    Disqualifications..17

    Breed Bans 18

Chapter 2: Where are Service Dogs Allowed?

    Places Covered under ADA Law...19

    Service Dogs in School...21

    Service Dogs at Work...21

    Service Dogs in Housing..22

    Service Dogs on Airplanes...23

    Scam Alert..24

Chapter 3: Your Rights and Responsibilities

    Know your Rights...26

    Your Responsibilities..27

    Documentation...28

Chapter 4: Service Dog Gear and Equipment

    Uniform 29

    Leash/Tether/Harness 30

    Booties 32

Chapter 5: Are You Ready to Begin Public Access Training?

    Essential Behavior 33

    Questionnaire: Are We Ready for Public Access Training? 35

    Public Access Readiness Evaluation Form 36

Chapter 6: Proofing and Generalization

    What is Generalization? 37

    Training Procedure Tips 38

    Proofing Worksheet 40

Chapter 7: Watch for Signs of Stress

    Stress Signals 41

    Stress Management 41

    Learn to Recognize Signs of Stress 42

    How can I help prevent or relieve my service dog's stress? 43

    Stress Evaluation 45

Chapter 8: How to Get Started

    Pet-friendly Locations 47

    Back to Phase I 48

    First Public Access Outing 49

    Your Markers 50

Chapter 9: Essential Tests

- AKC Canine Good Citizen and Beyond 51
- The Canine Good Citizen program 51
- Beyond the CGC 52
- ADI Public Access Test 53
- Task Foundation Training: Pass 54
- Public Access Practice Exam 55

Chapter 10: Challenges

- Access Challenges 65
- Dealing with People 66
- Your Role as the Educator 68
- Fake and Undertrained Service Dogs 69
- Role Playing Activity: The Things People Say 71

Chapter 11: Taking Action

- Filing a Title II Complaint 73
- Filing a Title III Complaint 76
- Resources 78
- Sample Complaint Letter 79

Chapter 12: Training Lessons

- Task Foundations: Harness Training 82
- A Personal Story 83
- Get Dressed (Harness) 87
- Target Stick 88
- Auto Check-in/Long Focus 89
- Leave-it 91

- Send Dog Out 92
- Pick up the Leash 93
- Under 94
- Find an Exit 95
- Circle Around and Got your 6 97
- Retrieve Items from Store Shelf 99
- Place Item in Basket 100
- Give Credit Card to Cashier 101
- Push Elevator Button 104
- About the Final Public Access Examination 108
- Your Final Exam 109
- Rules of the Helping Paws Final Public Access Examination 110
- Final Exam 111
- Scoring 117

Chapter 13: Worksheets

- Public Access Hours Log 122
- Public Access Practice Journal 126
- Task Training Tracker 131
- Public Access Training Overview 135
- Training Step Planning Tool 139
- Sample Letter to Request Permission to Train an SDiT in an Establishment..143
- Agreement Attesting to the level of training for reluctant establishments 145

PUBLIC ACCESS PREREQUISITES

Before you begin public access training, your dog should be reliable in (at least) the following cues. *Reliable* means the dog performs the cue 90% of the time at home and in pet-friendly establishments where you have practiced training.

- [ ] **NAME/WATCH**
- [ ] **SIT**
- [ ] **DOWN**
- [ ] **LONG DOWN/SPOT/STAY**
- [ ] **FOCUSED HEEL**
- [ ] **COME**
- [ ] **RELIEVE ON CUE**
- [ ] **LEAVE-IT**
- [ ] **UNDER (CHAIR OR TABLE)**
- [ ] **AT LEAST 1 TASK**

IMPORTANT VOCABULARY

If you have not read the other books in the Training your own Service Dog: The Complete Guide Series, some of the words I use may not make sense. I will list a couple of them below.

RELIABLE AT 90%

This statement refers to the point where a dog is able to follow a cue 9 out of 10 times or 90% of the time. At this point you are able to move to the next step.

LESSON TRAINING SEQUENCE

My program for balancing training with play and rest breaks for the dog to avoid burnout and loss of motivation. The program is in the front of this book.

SHAPING

Training a behavior by rewarding tiny steps towards the final behavior. As each step is mastered the reward is withheld until the dog offers a closer attempt at the final behavior being trained.

SDIT

Service Dog in Training

PROOFING

practicing a behavior in different environments and situations, until your dog generalizes the desired behavior and can do it anywhere, even with distractions.

GENERALIZATION

When a dog can apply a concept to many situations. (Dogs do not do this very well naturally).

PLATFORM TRAINNG

The *platform* gives your dog a concrete boundary (the edge of the platform). Arguably the fastest way to teach "stay" and other cues.

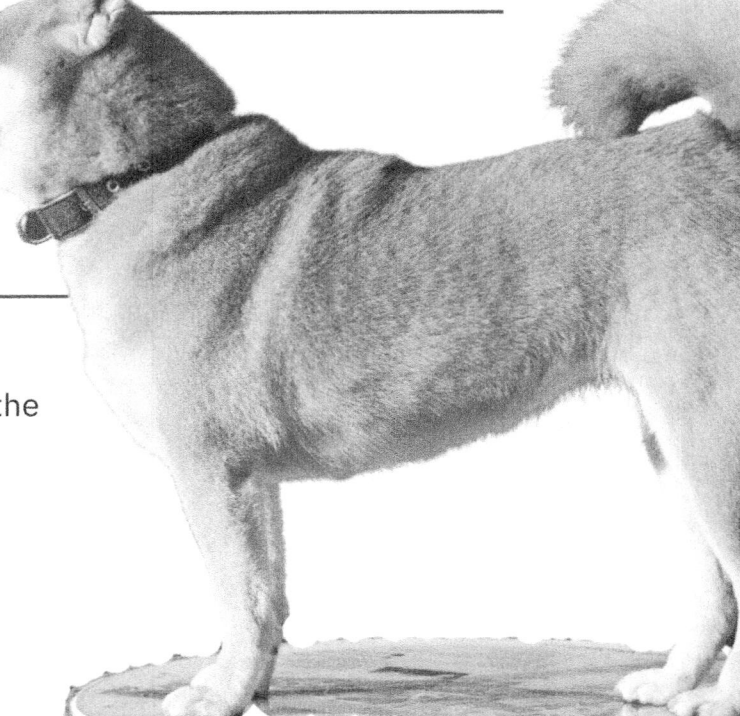

Welcome to Volume IV, the next level of training your service dog! Congratulations on the progress you have made to make it this far.

By now you have read Volume I and worked through the lessons in Volume II, If you are raising a puppy, hopefully you have read Volume III as well.

This program consists of solidifying the behaviors learned in Volumes I and II, as well as setting the foundation for task training in order to prepare for public access.

At the end of the program, you can take the included Public Access Examination. Practice as many times as you need with the practice exam in week three of this workbook.

I have included a couple of lessons from previous volumes, I apologize to those of you who have already read these lessons in my other books in this series. The reason they are included is for one of two reasons.

The first reason is that it is important enough to be repeated. The second reason it might have been repeated is that some of the material would not make sense unless you read the other books in the series and I do not want anyone confused or left behind.

I have also included only a couple of the foundation behaviors that are the basis of all tasks. The main foundation behaviors are targeting, retrieve, tug, stand/stay, and paws up.

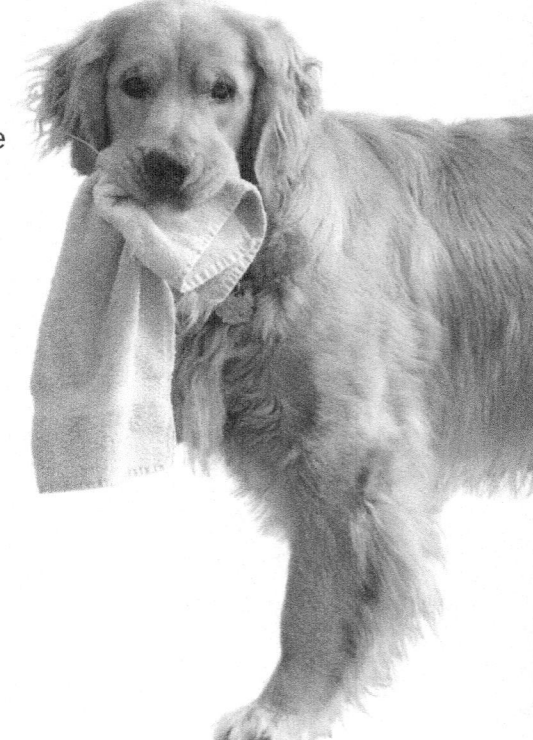

I have included targeting in almost every volume because targeting is the foundation of so many behaviors. These foundation behaviors will be covered in a short but informative volume that covers all of the foundation behaviors and will actually be released before the (much-awaited) Task Training book.

Because I decided to publish the Foundation Skills book, I decided not to put many of the foundation behaviors in the Public Access volume.

However, I urge you to get the next book in this series on foundation behaviors right away, as these are skills you will want to be working on to prepare for task training.

Mega Learn SYSTEM

Follow my 4-phase training program for extremely reliable results.

The Mega Learn System works for all dogs, no matter their age, breed, or amount/type of previous training.

The important thing is to find what motivates your dog. What does your dog really like? Chicken, ham, bacon, cheese, hard-boiled eggs?

All dogs are at least somewhat motivated by food, especially their favorite food. After all, they need it to survive!

It is important to note that a finicky attitude can be fostered when a dog is free-fed (allowed to eat at will) or is fed high-value (favorite) foods without being asked to work for it.

> Once you find the reward(s) that your dog will work the hardest for, following the commandments you can begin each new behavior at phase one. If your dog "sort of knows how to sit" or "sometimes comes when called" you should start over using the Mega Learn System.

PHASE I
- On-leash
- High-value rewards to lure behavior
- Praise and reward every correct behavior
- No verbal cue
- No distractions

PHASE II
- On-leash
- Praise and reward every correct behavior
- Add verbal cue (spoken BEFORE the physical cue/lure)
- No distractions

PHASE III
- Leash attached
- Praise correct behavior
- Verbal cue THEN hand signal
- Intermittent (varied) reward
- No distractions

PHASE IV
- Off-leash
- Intermittent reward
- Verbal cue OR hand signal
- Begin to remove rewards
- No distractions

- Move from one phase to another when your dog is performing the behavior reliably 100% of the time)
- When you master Phase IV, go back to phase I and add distractions, duration and distance gradually

LESSON TRAINING SEQUENCE

- Follow this sequence for teaching **new** behaviors
- ALWAYS end on a positive note by asking your dog to do something he/she knows and can perform
- Phases 1-4 are trained with NO distractions
- ALWAYS reward your dog with a walk or playtime after a training session

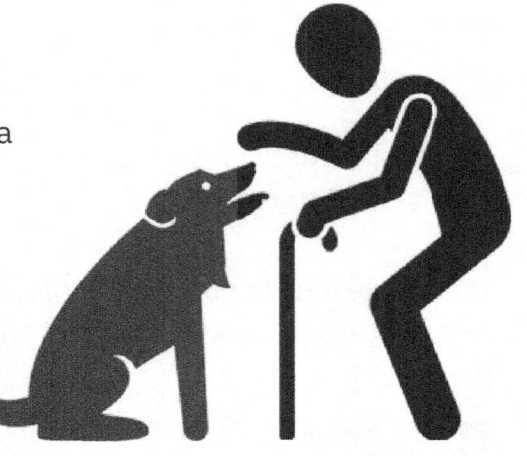

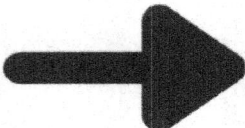

Segment #1
10x Repetitions

→ • Give your dog a 1-3 minute break

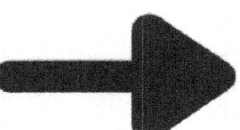

Segment #2
10x Repetitions of the same command

→
- Give your dog a 1-3 minute break
- Give some affection or play time

- End session on with a successful execution of a behavior to help build confidence

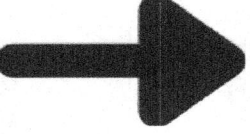

Segment #3
10x Repetitions of the same command

→ • Take your dog for a walk or have some play time doing something your dog enjoys for 10 minutes or so

Repeat this sequence 3 or more times a day for new cues

CHAPTER 1:
WHAT QUALIFIES MY DOG AS A SERVICE DOG?

The ADA defines a Service Dog as:
"Any dog that is individually trained to do work or perform tasks for the benefit of an individual with a disability, including a physical; sensory; psychiatric; intellectual; or other mental disability."

The definition also states:
"The work or task a dog has been trained to provide must be directly related to the person's disability. Dogs whose sole function is to provide comfort or emotional support do not qualify as service animals under the ADA."

The ADA defines a person with a "disability" as:
"A person who has a physical or mental impairment that substantially limits one or more major life activity"

The ADA defines a disability different than other laws, such as Social Security. Under the ADA, disability is a legal term rather than a medical term.

SERVICE DOG-IN-TRAINING VS. FULL-FLEDGED SERVICE DOG

COMMON MYTHS AND CONFUSION

It seems that different opinions exist on when exactly an *SDiT* graduates to full service-dog status.

I read everything I can get my hands on regarding service dogs and laws that cover them so I can keep my books up-to-date as much as possible. I have seen some pretty wild opinions from service dog organizations that are not listed anywhere in the law.

Statements such as:
- Service dogs must be trained in 3 tasks
- Psychiatric service dogs need a doctor's note for public access
- Service dogs are REQUIRED to pass the Public Access Test

Nowhere in the ADA law does it say anything about a specific number of tasks that must be trained prior to public access being permitted.

As far as the Public Access Test; I highly recommend that service dog teams should pass the public access test. After all, you have worked really hard, and passing the test is the ultimate success.
Aside from the satisfaction of acing the test, service dog handlers generally seem to hold themselves and their dogs to a higher standard of training and etiquette.

While it is generally accepted that the public access test is part of public access, it is not a requirement as of when this book was published. This may change in the near future partially due to abuse of the law. (Discussed later in this book).

- That ONLY trained tasks are recognized and something a dog does naturally would not count as work

This statement is listed in the law, however, I think certain things a service dog may learn to do on its own certainly fall within the parameters of the law.

I feel there is a great deal of confusion surrounding tasks and what is called "work".

In both *work* and *tasks*, a dog responds to a cue. When a cue is intentionally given by the handler (verbal, hand signal) for a behavior that was trained, and the dog responds, s/he is performing a task.

When the dog responds to a cue from a handler that is not intentional (handler slumps over and the dog goes for help), or from the environment (Guide dog blocks handler from walking out in traffic when he sees cars coming) would be considered work.

Work, in the context of service dogs, from what I understand may have been trained initially but is often something dogs learn to do on their own.

I trained a service dog team early on in my service dog training days that are would be a perfect example.

Bailey was a rescued Chocolate Lab and her handler, Meaghan, had a number of serious health issues. One of her conditions caused frequent, uncontrolled seizures.

When I matched Meaghan with Bailey, I trained her for seizure response (tasks such as getting help; bringing a blanket, and making an emergency call using a cell phone I modified based on plans a service dog trainer in Britain had shared on the internet, etc.) I did not provide a guaranteed seizure alert dog.

I knew there was a possibility that she could learn to communicate to Meaghan and warn of an oncoming seizure, but that Meaghan would need to pay attention to Bailey's subtle behavior and look for a pattern to occur of how she acted BEFORE the seizure. I also knew this might be difficult because after having a seizure, most people are pretty foggy. Also, I encourage family members to observe the dog and recall any behaviors they noticed prior to a seizure. However, if one lives alone this does not work as well.

Long story short, Bailey DID begin to alert Meaghan effectively on her own, before every seizure she had. Meaghan did not teach her this behavior; she simply learned to interpret Bailey's own alert system.

My point is that this was not an intentionally trained task. This was something Bailey taught herself and an example of teamwork and a relationship based on communication.

It is my opinion that this example of "work" is just as important as a task that was trained and that the ADA description can be confusing in that regard.

How about this one:
- According to one airline, a service dog should be at least 4 months old

Four months old? I know for certain that is NOT in the law! I am pretty certain four months is way too young to be expected to handle the responsibility of being a full service dog.

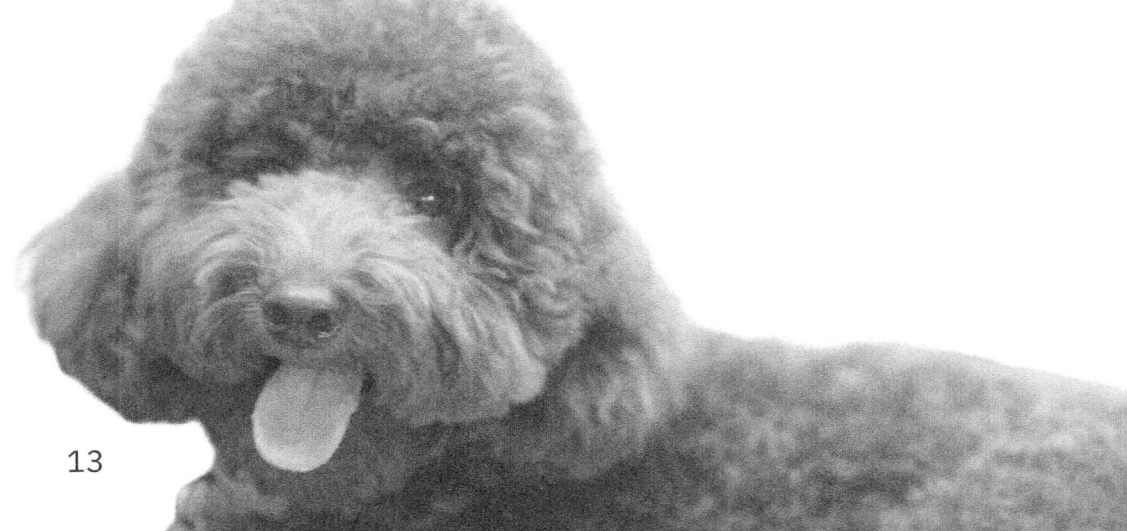

SO, WHEN DOES AN SDIT BECOME A SERVICE DOG?

While the law does not specifically state the guidelines I am about to mention, I think it is generally agreed upon within the service dog community that to become a full-fledged Service Dog your team will have mastered the following:

- Service dogs are not only completely housebroken but will relieve themselves on cue

- Be 95% or above in reliability in basic obedience (name/watch/focus; sit; down; stay; come; heel; leave-it; settle etc.)

- Is able to ignore people and other animals and focus on the handler

- Has learned or is quickly learning one or more tasks and/or work directly related to the handler's disability

- Has close to 120 hours or more of service dog specific training documented

- Has passed the Public Access Test, although this is still optional

- Is able to settle down in public and lie down under a table or otherwise out of the way of other people

- Knows not to seek attention or sniff people or merchandise

All of these milestones are much easier to reach when you can take your dog into public places during training. In states where an SDiT is not allowed public access while in training, you will have to be creative.

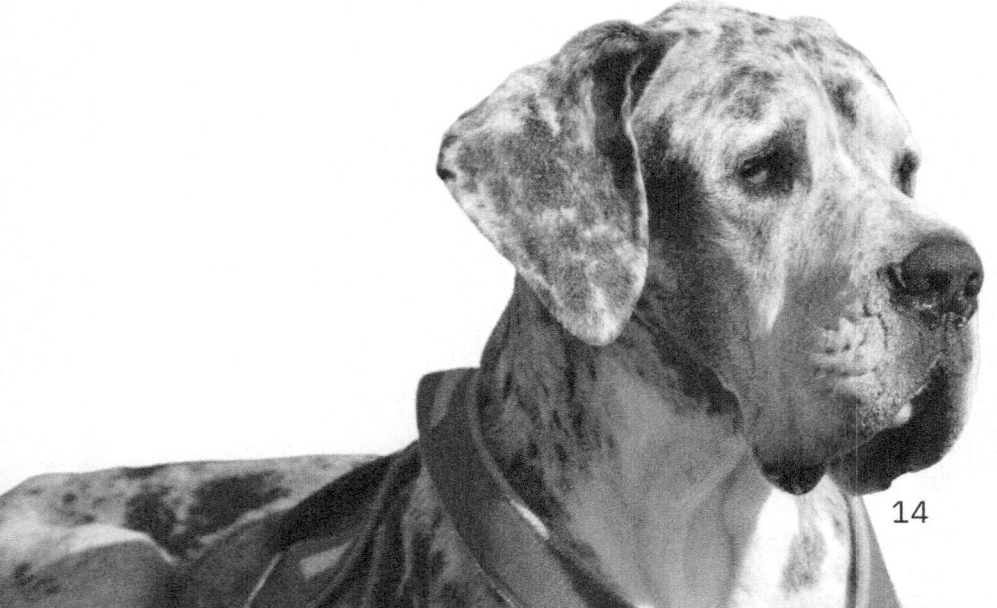

STATE LAWS

Federal ADA law does not cover service dogs in training (SDiT). You must determine whether your state mentions SDiT or not. Not every state in the US covers your Service Dog while it is in training and some states mention SDiT but have additional stipulations handlers must abide by.

Here is a brief list of states and whether or not they mention SDiT or not. This list was current at the time this book was published.

STATES THAT DO NOT MENTION PUBLIC ACCESS FOR SERVICE DOGS IN TRAINING
- Hawaii
- South Dakota
- Wyoming

STATES THAT ALLOW PUBLIC ACCESS TO SERVICE DOGS IN TRAINING
- Alabama
- Arizona
- Colorado
- Connecticut
- Delaware
- Florida
- Illinois
- Indiana
- Iowa
- Louisiana
- Maine
- Maryland
- Massachusetts
- Michigan (2022)
- Minnesota
- Mississippi
- Nevada
- New Hampshire
- New Jersey
- New Mexico
- Ohio
- Oregon
- Pennsylvania
- Rhode Island
- South Carolina
- Utah
- Vermont

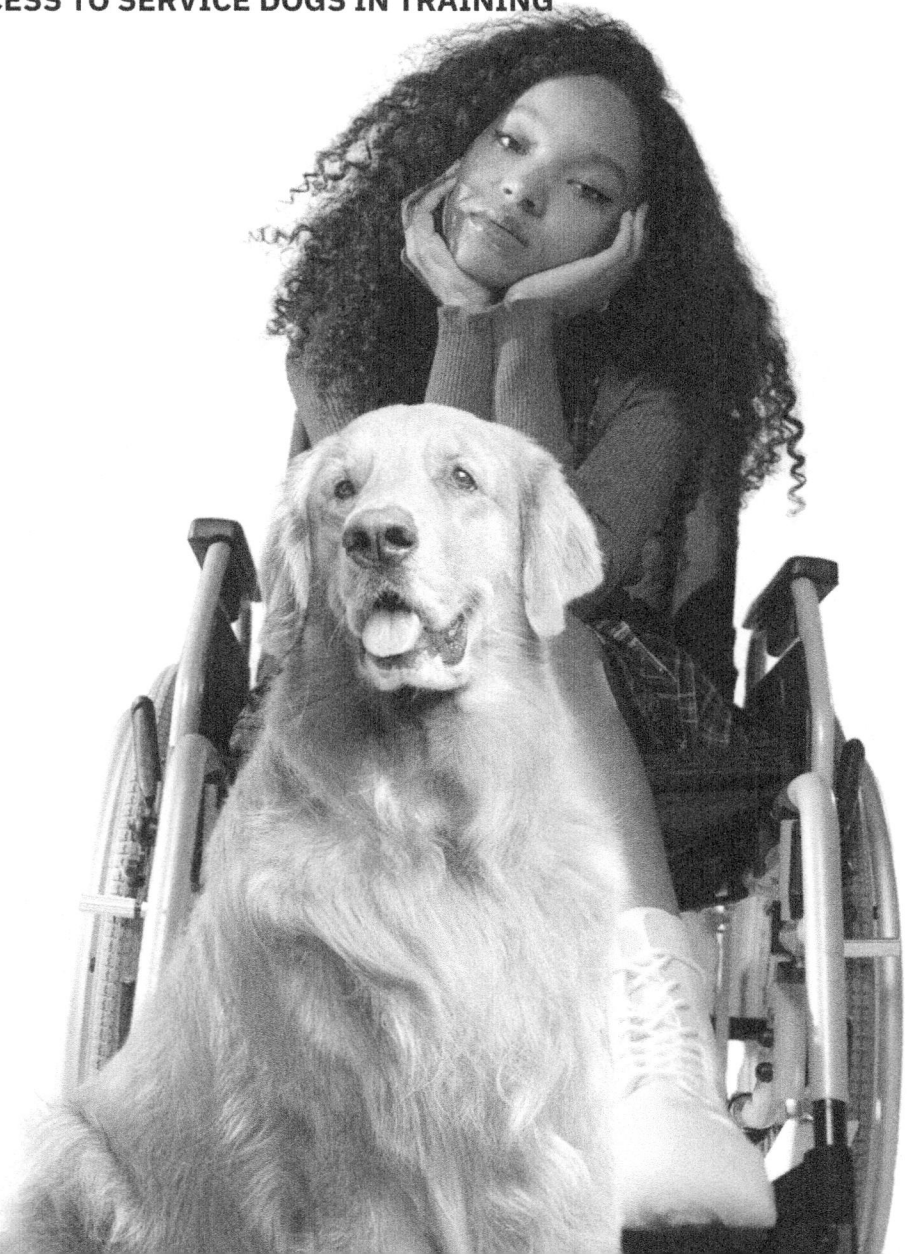

STATES THAT ALLOW PUBLIC ACCESS TO SERVICE DOGS IN TRAINING WITH ADDITIONAL STIPULATIONS

Additional stipulations may include trainers being certified or accredited by a recognized school, required to wear a vest from a recognized school or that is a certain color, or "tagged" by the county clerk as a service dog. If you live in one of the states in this list, make sure you do some further research into what the law states.

- Alaska
- California
- Georgia
- Idaho
- Kansas
- Kentucky
- Missouri
- Montana
- Nebraska
- New York
- North Carolina
- North Dakota
- Oklahoma
- Tennessee
- Texas
- Virginia
- Washington
- West Virginia
- Wisconsin

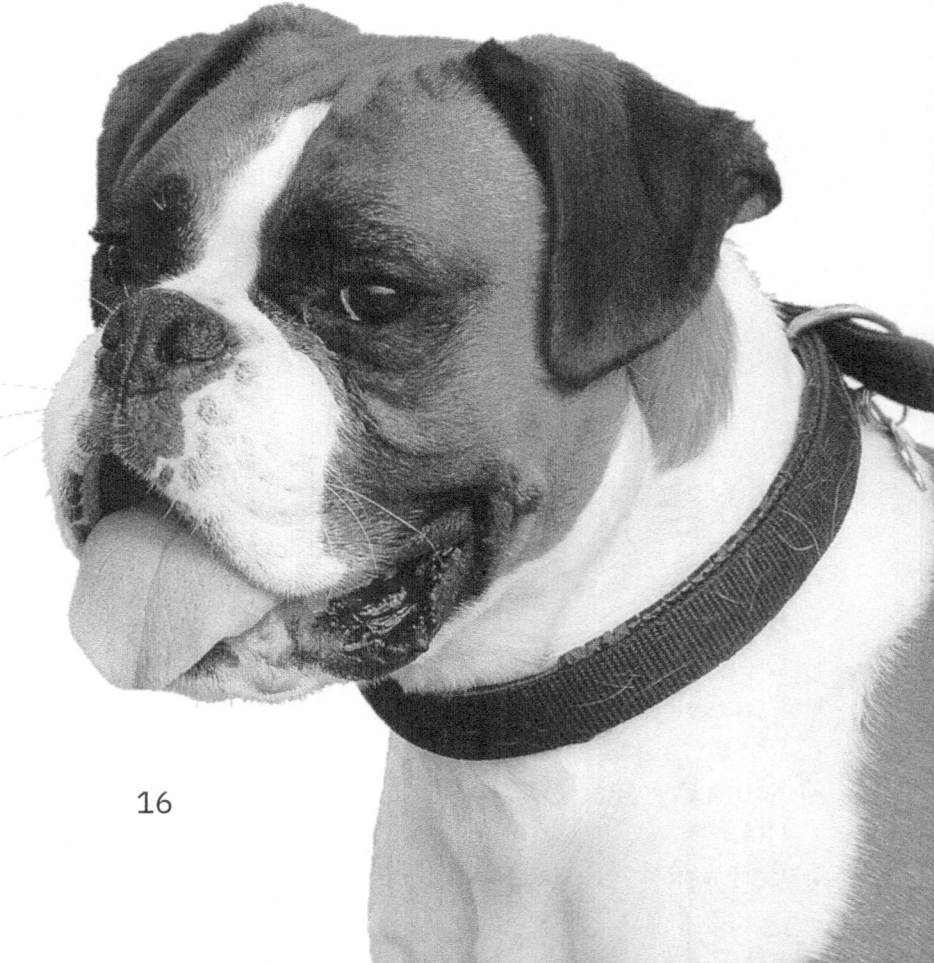

DISQUALIFICATIONS

Under Federal ADA law, a service dog team cannot be excluded from a business due to:

- Size of service dog
- Breed of service dog
- A "No-pets policy"
- Allergies
- Fear of dogs
- Not providing "papers" or other proof
- Not wearing a vest
- The sole reason being that it is a food establishment

A service dog team CAN be excluded from a business due to:

- A service dog not being housebroken
- Being disruptive (i.e. barking unless it is part of an alert task)
- Aggression of any sort
- Not being "under control" if the handler does not take reasonable action to control the dog
- Not being leashed/harnessed unless being tethered would interfere with the service dog's trained task and the dog must remain under the control of the handler
- The handler being unable/unwilling to answer the appropriate questions when asked or stating the dog's primary task is emotional support

If a service dog is excluded from an establishment, the handler should still be offered services without the presence of the dog.

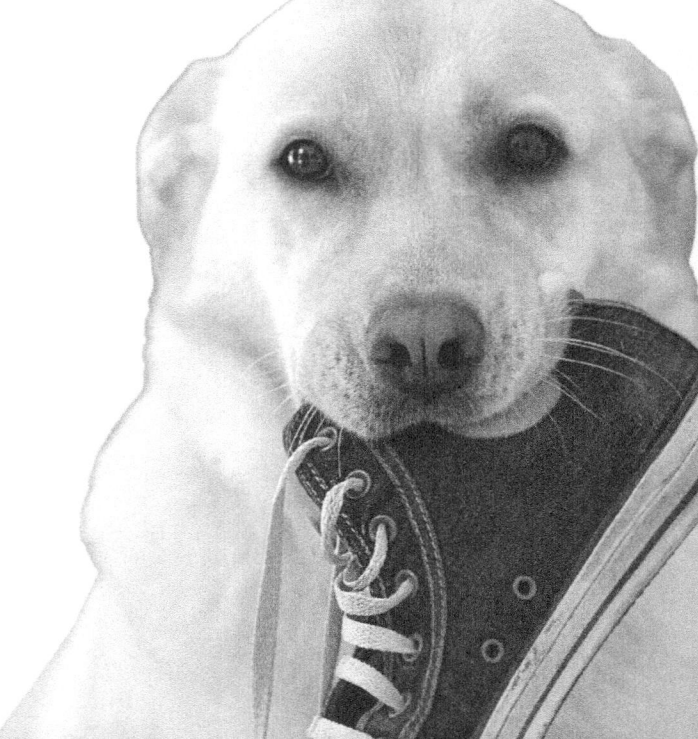

BREED BANS

Breed bans do not apply to service dogs. However, you might want to think about using a so-called "controversial" breed that has stigma attached to them such as a Pit Bull. Other Bully types, Rottweilers and Dobermans can also bring you unwanted attention. The reason for this is many people are afraid of them and you will encounter more access challenges.

I know this from experience because I ran an organization called Bulldogs for Soldiers. I raised and trained Olde English Bulldogges and placed them with veterans suffering from PTSD.

My dogs were carefully selected and bred for health and especially temperament. They looked fierce but were very good-natured.

In general, service dogs attract a good deal of attention anyway. When a service dog is of a certain breed, they can attract more attention and it is not always good attention.

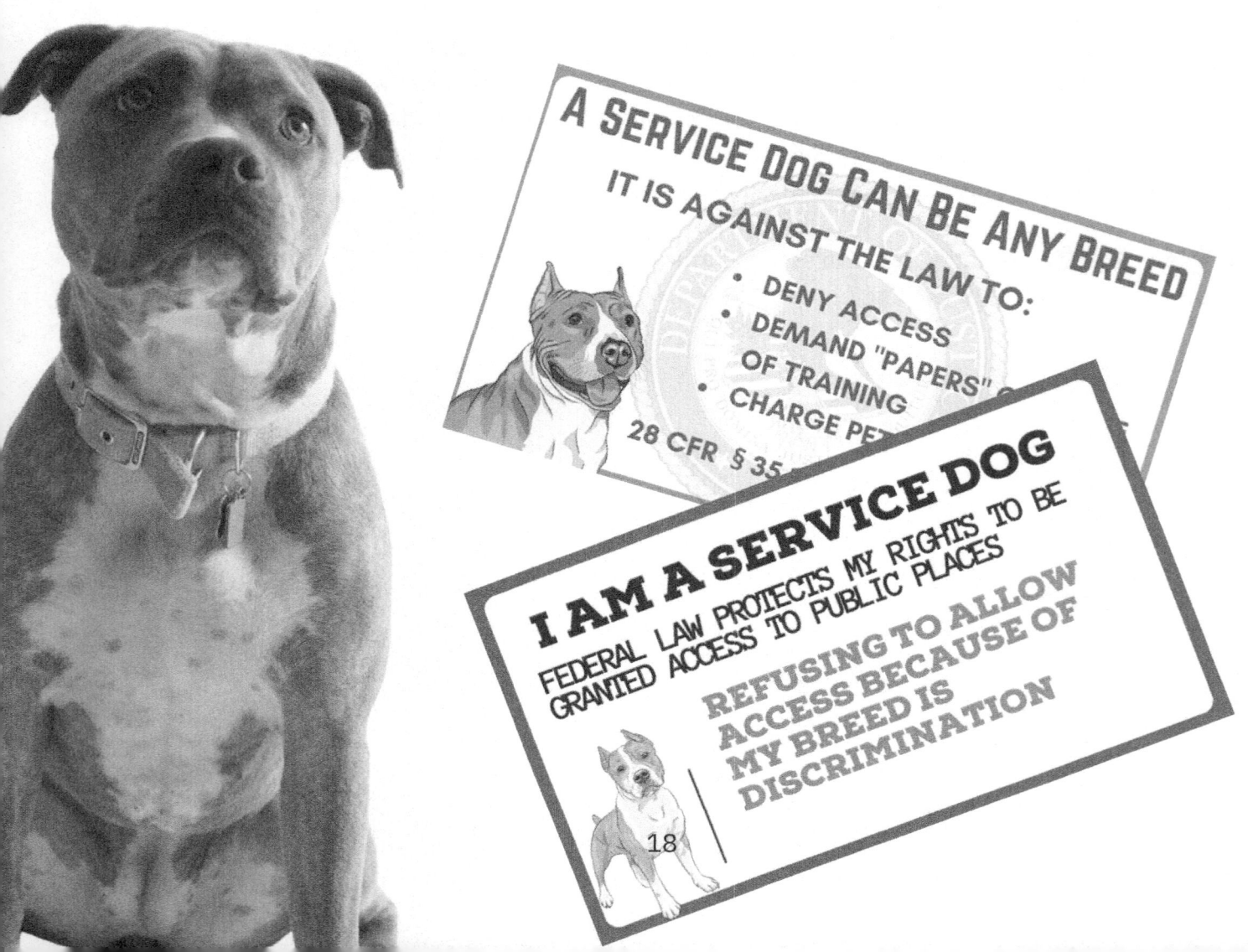

CHAPTER 2:
WHERE ARE SERVICE DOGS ALLOWED?

PLACES COVERED UNDER ADA LAW

Note: The ADA does NOT cover Service Dogs in Training (SDiT) in the law. The following information applies to Service Dogs only. Many states do have laws that refer to SDiT, so check state and local laws to determine if your SDiT is covered.

"The ADA requires State and local government agencies, businesses, and non-profit organizations (covered entities) that provide goods or services to the public to make "reasonable modifications" in their policies, practices, or procedures when necessary to accommodate people with disabilities. The service animal rules fall under this general principle.
Accordingly, entities that have a 'no pets' policy generally must modify the policy to allow service animals into their facilities."
—ADA website

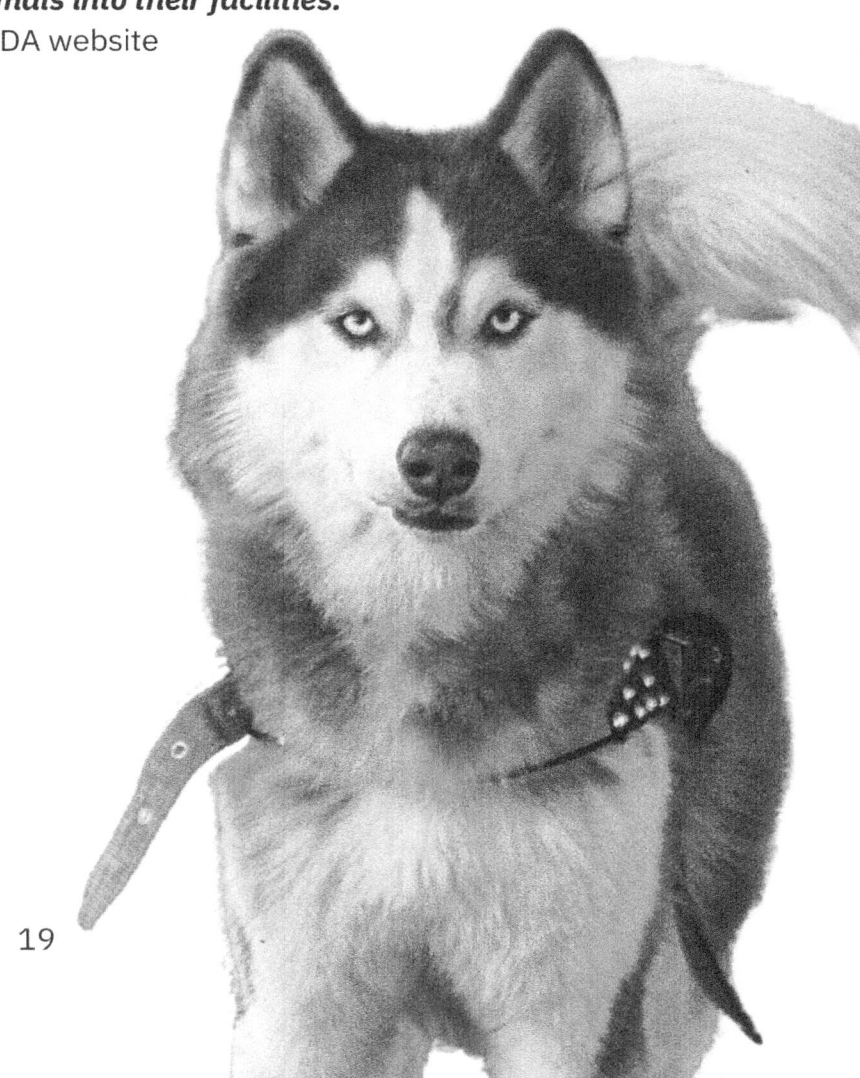

TITLE III OF THE ADA COVERS:

- Hotels/motels
- Hospitals* and Doctor offices
- Places serving food or drink (restaurants and bars)
- Theaters and other places of entertainment
- Auditoriums
- Retail stores and shopping centers
- Service providers
- Airports, Bus, and Train stations
- Museums/galleries
- Amusement parks
- Social services centers (day care for children or adults, food banks, homeless shelters)
- Gyms
- Taxis and other ground transportation
- Educational testing sites

While service dogs are permitted in hospitals, certain areas would be off limits such as operating rooms and burn units if the presence of the dog might pose a risk of infection. (These areas do not allow access to the general public anyway).

TITLE III OF THE ADA DOES NOT COVER:

- State and local government programs, services, and activities (Title II)
- Employment (Title I)
- Private clubs and establishments
- Religious organizations including places of worship, unless facilities are also leased to hold public events
- AMTRAK (Title II)
- Housing (HUD)
- Aircraft (ACAA/DOT)
- Schools (Section 504/Title II)

SERVICE DOGS IN SCHOOL

Service dogs are allowed in school, but there are many factors to be considered. In elementary, middle, and high school a service dog will be allowed as long as the student is able to manage the animal and the dog cannot be aggressive, is housebroken, and is under the control of the handler.

The school is required to make accommodations such as making sure an accessible place to allow the dog to eliminate exists but is not required to provide someone to help manage the animal.

Schools may request documents such as proof of rabies vaccination but it is not required that you provide this.

At colleges and universities, a service dog is covered under Title II. Housing in dormitories is covered by HUD under the Fair Housing act rather than the ADA.

SERVICE DOGS AT WORK

Employees are covered under Title I of the ADA law. Title I requires employers to make "reasonable accommodations" for employees. This means that an employee must request a reasonable accommodation from an employer.

An accommodation is considered reasonable as long as it does not create undue hardship or pose a threat.

Examples of "reasonable accommodations" may include altering the No Pets Policy and altering work schedules for other employees who are allergic to dogs.

SERVICE DOGS IN HOUSING

The Federal Fair Housing Act covers service animals and Emotional Support Animals in rentals and dormitories.

Assistance animals, including ESA, are under a different legal classification when it comes to rental tenants. You cannot be charged pet fees and are not subject to pet restrictions. ***A Service Dog is not a pet.*** Breed and weight restrictions do not apply.

Emotional Support Animals Only:
In order to request a reasonable accommodation for Emotional Support Animals (which are not necessarily dogs) you should provide the landlord with a document from your doctor/therapist that states that you have a disabling condition and why it is necessary for you to have this animal for emotional support.

FFHA DOES NOT APPLY IN CERTAIN SITUATIONS, INCLUDING:

- Rental dwellings of four or fewer units, where one unit is occupied by the owner
- Single-family homes sold or rented by the owner without the use of a broker
- Housing owned by private clubs or religious organizations that restrict occupancy in housing units to their members
- As long as your disability request is true and there is no indication that your request would cause hardship, landlords must comply. You cannot be charged pet fees but you are responsible for any damages caused by your service dog or emotional support animal
- In the case a landlord refuses to comply you have the right to request a government agency look into your complaint that you have been discriminated against.
- File a discrimination complaint with HUD and check to see if your state has a government agency that investigates discrimination claims. If so, file a complaint directly with your state as well

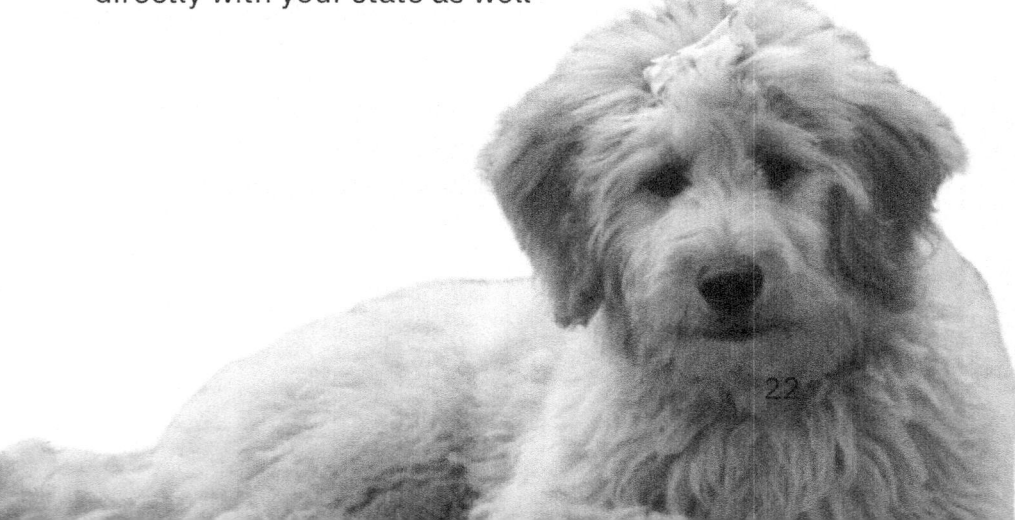

SERVICE DOGS ON AIRPLANES

The ADA covers the airport but the actual aircraft is covered under the Air Carrier Access Act (ACAA). Emotional Support Animals used to be covered under these guidelines, but amendments made to the law in 2020 now cover only service dogs. Service dogs in training are not specifically mentioned.

- Airlines are required to transport service dogs within the US as well as to and from the US
- Airlines can deny transporting a service dog to a US territory or country that prohibits entry to the dog.

AIRLINES CAN ALSO DENY TRANSPORT IF:

- It violates safety regulations (i.e. too large to fit in the cabin)
- It poses a direct threat to the safety of others
- It causes a significant disruption at the gate or in the cabin
- If the airline requires DOT forms to be submitted and the handler fails to submit them

Service dog handlers may be required to fill out either a form that attests to the health and training of your service dog and/or a form that attests that your service dog will either not relieve itself or relieve itself in a sanitary manner on flights lasting 8 hours or longer.

If you feel you have been discriminated against during your air travel you have the right to file a complaint with the DOT.

A consumer report can be filed online https://www.transportation.gov/individuals/aviation-consumer-protection/service-animals or by mail.

You may contact DOT by phone at 202-366-2220. However, in order for a case to be processed as a complaint, it must be submitted in writing.

Send your correspondence to the below address:

Office of Aviation Consumer Protection
U.S. Department of Transportation
1200 New Jersey Avenue, SE
Washington, DC 20590

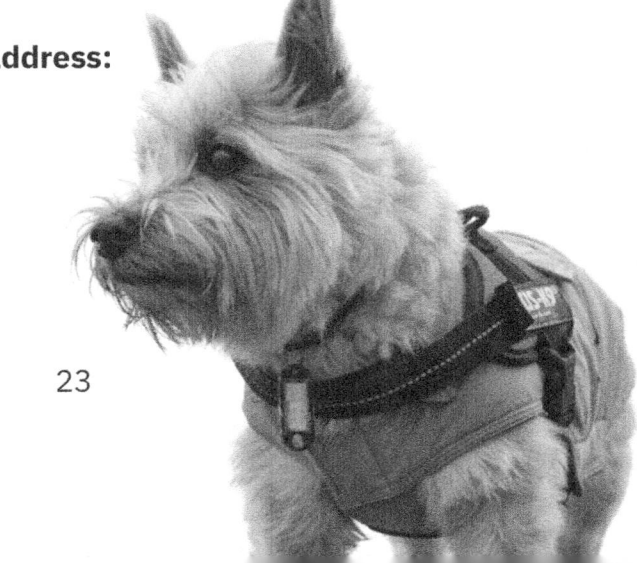

Service dogs are not required by law to wear a vest or carry ID when in public.

A service dog is also not required to be "certified". In fact, there is not even a certification in the US that is federally recognized at this point!

Some programs that train service dogs may certify dogs through their program, but this means nothing as far as far as ADA law is concerned.

There are several online companies that will try and sell you "certification" or "registration" papers for a hefty fee. These are a scam.

It is optional to register with one of these registries, most of them will allow you to register your service dog in their database for free, but then they hit you with a service dog package with a vest and "papers". They often make it seem like you have to pay the fee and get the registration papers so your dog is legit.
DON'T FALL FOR IT!

First of all, no one can "certify" a dog as a service dog if they didn't participate in the training or at least have done some sort of evaluation of the dog's training skills.

This is a big problem in recent years because these dogs may misbehave and since the handler provided the proverbial "papers" everyone always illegally asks for, it makes businesses think that we must be required to carry "papers", which makes access challenges for us even more stressful.

When possible, I always dress my dog or a dog I am training. Any time I have not has resulted in an access challenge.

CHAPTER 3: YOUR RIGHTS AND RESPONSIBILITIES

"The Americans with Disabilities Act (ADA) was passed in 1990 and gives civil rights protections to individuals with disabilities similar to those provided to individuals on the basis of race, color, sex, national origin, age and religion. It works to break down barriers to employment, transportation, public accommodations, public services and telecommunications for people with disabilities."

—*The U.S. Department of Justice*

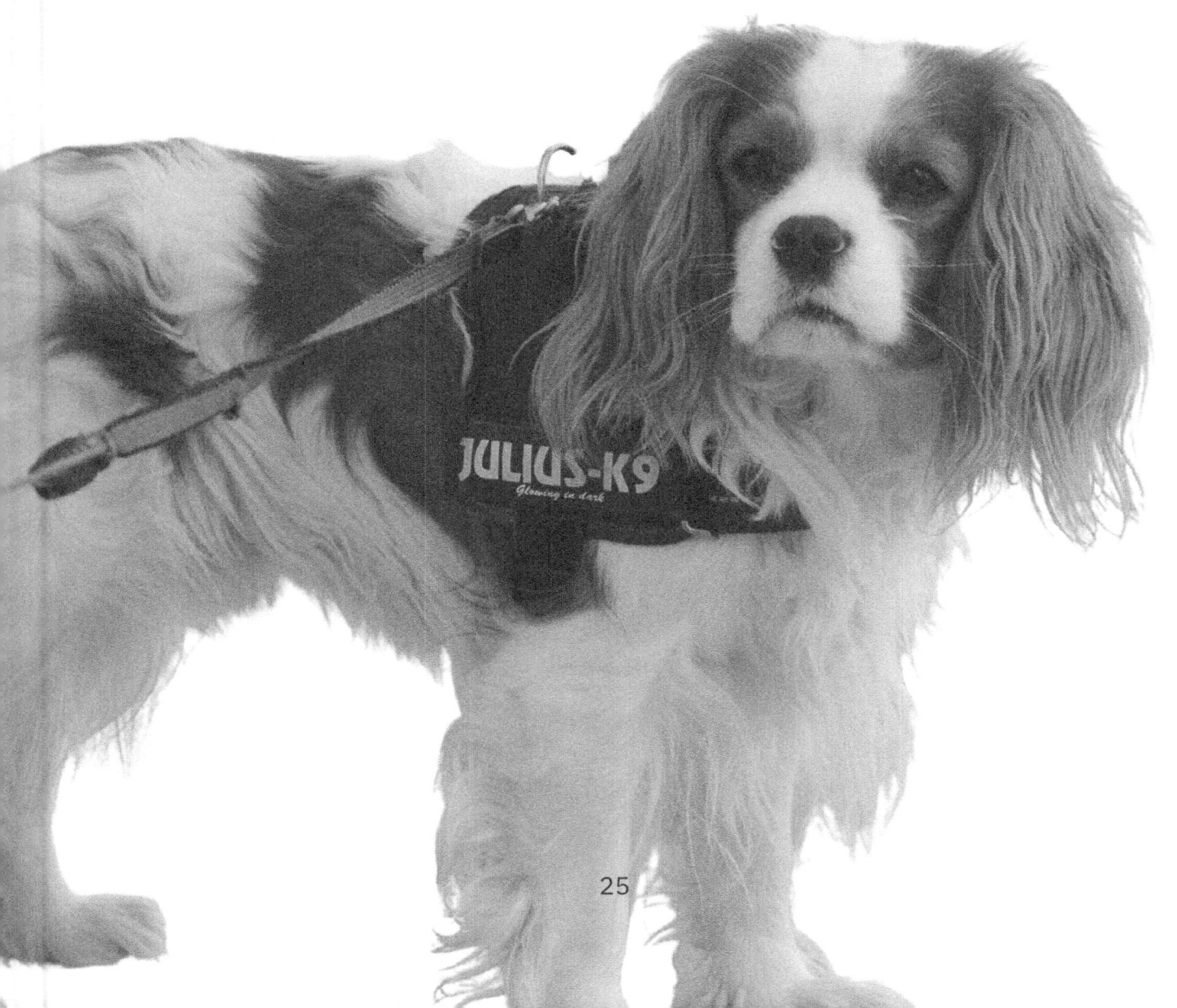

KNOW YOUR RIGHTS

It is important to note that people are covered under ADA law, not dogs.

• You have the right to be accompanied by your service dog, as long as your dog is well-behaved, trained, and clean. If your service dog was to be excluded from an establishment due to behavior, you still have the right to receive goods or services without the presence of your dog

• You have the right to equal treatment. You should be treated the same as someone without a disability. If you are in an establishment with your service dog, you cannot be secluded from other people or excluded from any area the general public is allowed

• Allergies and fear of dogs are not valid reasons to exclude a service dog. The business is required to accommodate the needs of both parties in this case

• A "No Pets" policy does not apply to service dogs, even in a food establishment *(A service dog is not a pet)*

• You should not be charged extra or be required to pay pet fees. You are responsible for damages should any occur

• Businesses cannot ask you to provide proof of your disability or demonstrate your service dog's tasks

• Businesses cannot ask about your disability (with the exception of the allowed questions)

• You have the right to have more than one service dog as long as they are needed for a disability, trained to perform task(s) that mitigate your disability, and are under your control

• You have the right to train your own service dog

• You have the right to file a complaint if you feel you have been discriminated against

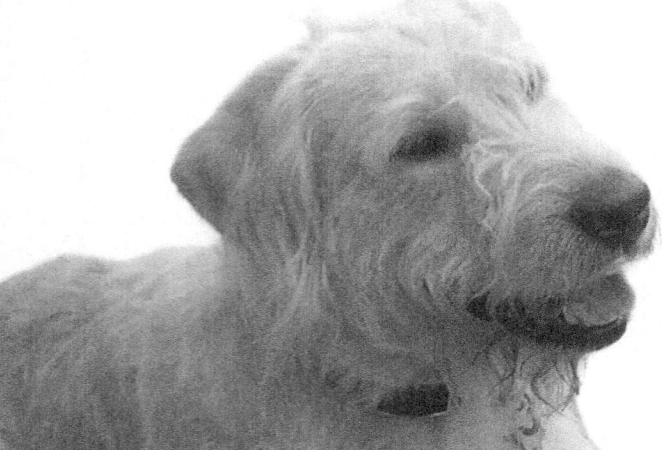

YOUR RESPONSIBILITIES

YOU ARE RESPONSIBLE FOR:

- Presenting your team in a professional manner

- Your service dog's behavior

- Damages caused by your service dog

- Maintaining the grooming and cleanliness of your service dog

- Cleaning up after your dog

- Presenting yourself and your service dog in a professional manner

- Keeping your service dog leashed, unless it would interfere with performing a task. In this case, your service dog must be under your control at all times

- Maintaining the training of your service dog

- The sole care of your service dog while in public

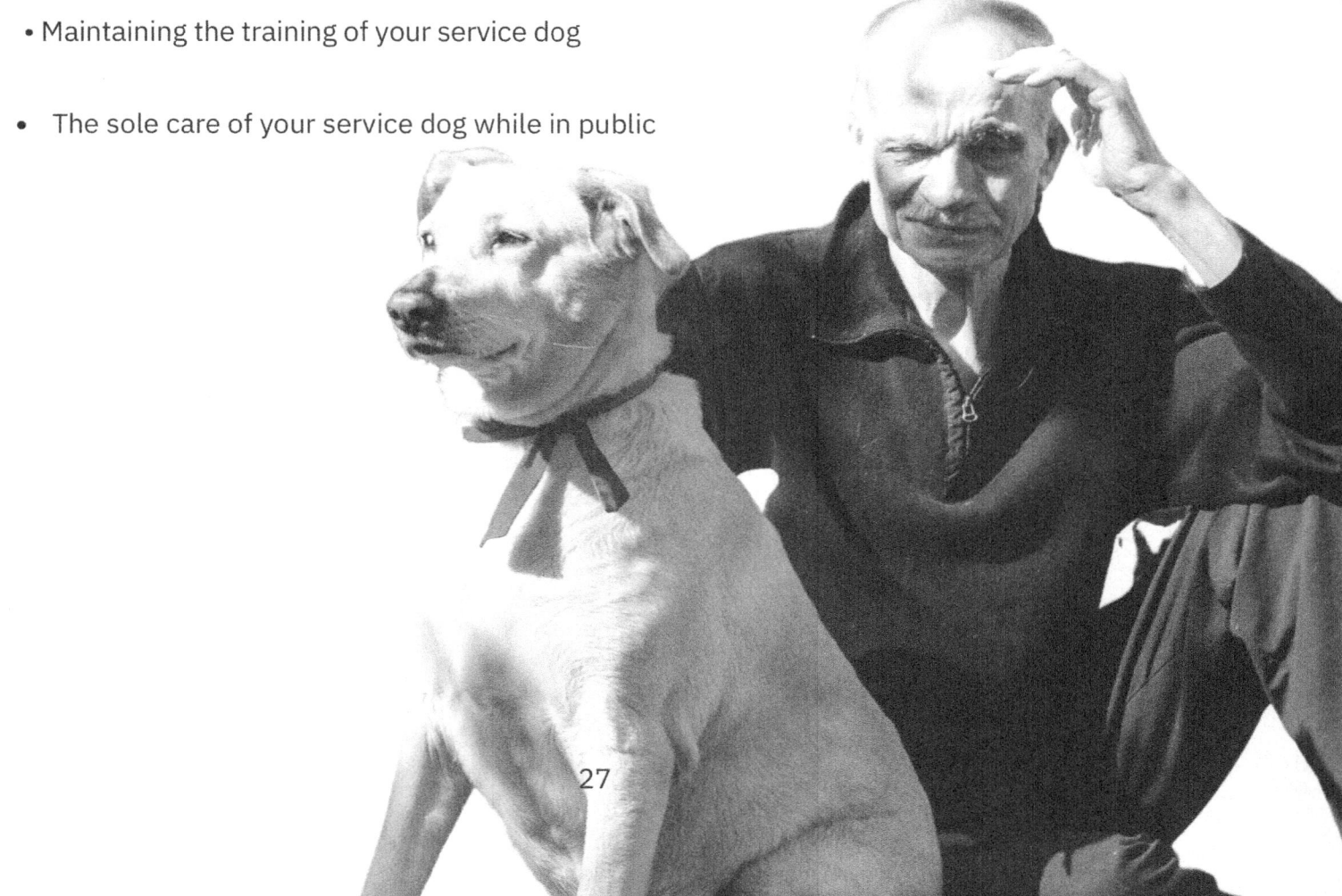

DOCUMENTATION

It is very important to document all of your training. Documentation is important in case you'll ever have to prove the extent of training your dog has.

If heaven forbid, you were ever to end up in court or mediation (on either side of the law) you will want your case to be airtight.

It is notoriously difficult for service dog handlers to prove their case without documentation that proves how much training a service dog has had prior to a court hearing. I recommend keeping a binder complete with any classes you have completed with your dog, awards and certificates such as S.T.A.R. Puppy and Canine Good Citizen certifications, training logs that document training hours, and training journals that give detailed information about training sessions.

Keep video footage of passing your Public Access Test.

Keeping this documentation is also extremely valuable so you can see the progress your team has made and where you need work.

You will find worksheets, logs, and different types of journals in this book as well as in Volume II to give you a variety of tools to use for documenting training. Choose which ones are most helpful and use them every time you train.

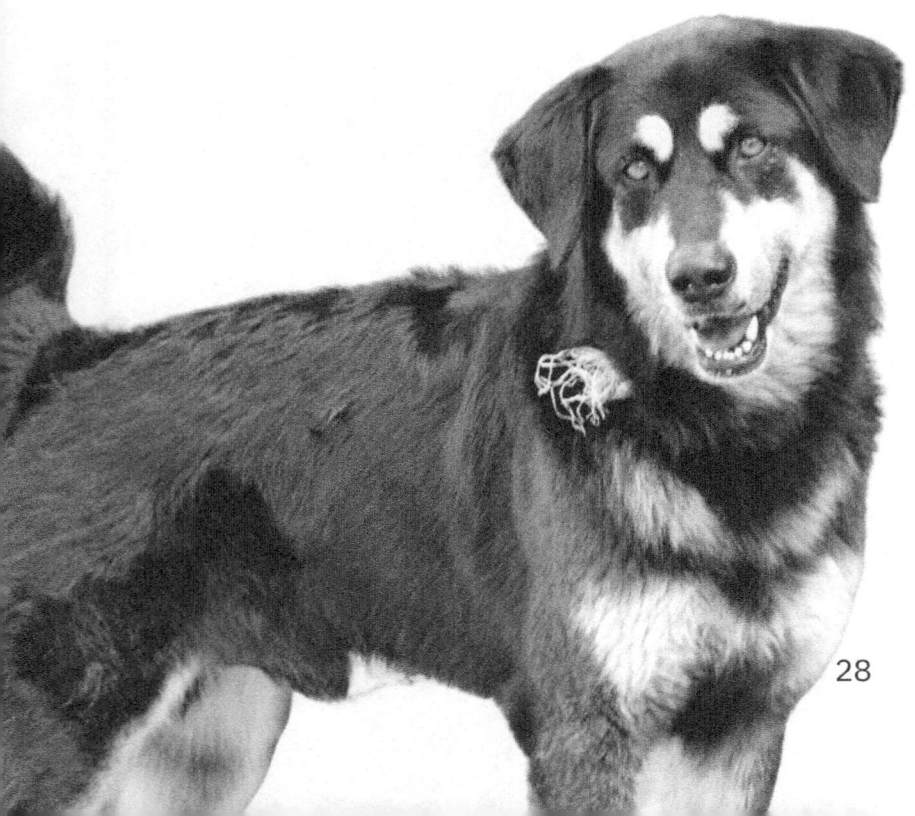

CHAPTER 4: SERVICE DOG EQUIPMENT AND GEAR

UNIFORM

Service dogs are not required by law to wear a vest or cape. However, most handlers choose to identify their service dog by outfitting them in some sort of uniform.

I find that I encounter far fewer access challenges when my dog is wearing a vest. I also found that dogs learn that putting their vest on means work and they get serious when I put it on.

I do not allow anyone, including family members, to pet them when they are in uniform.

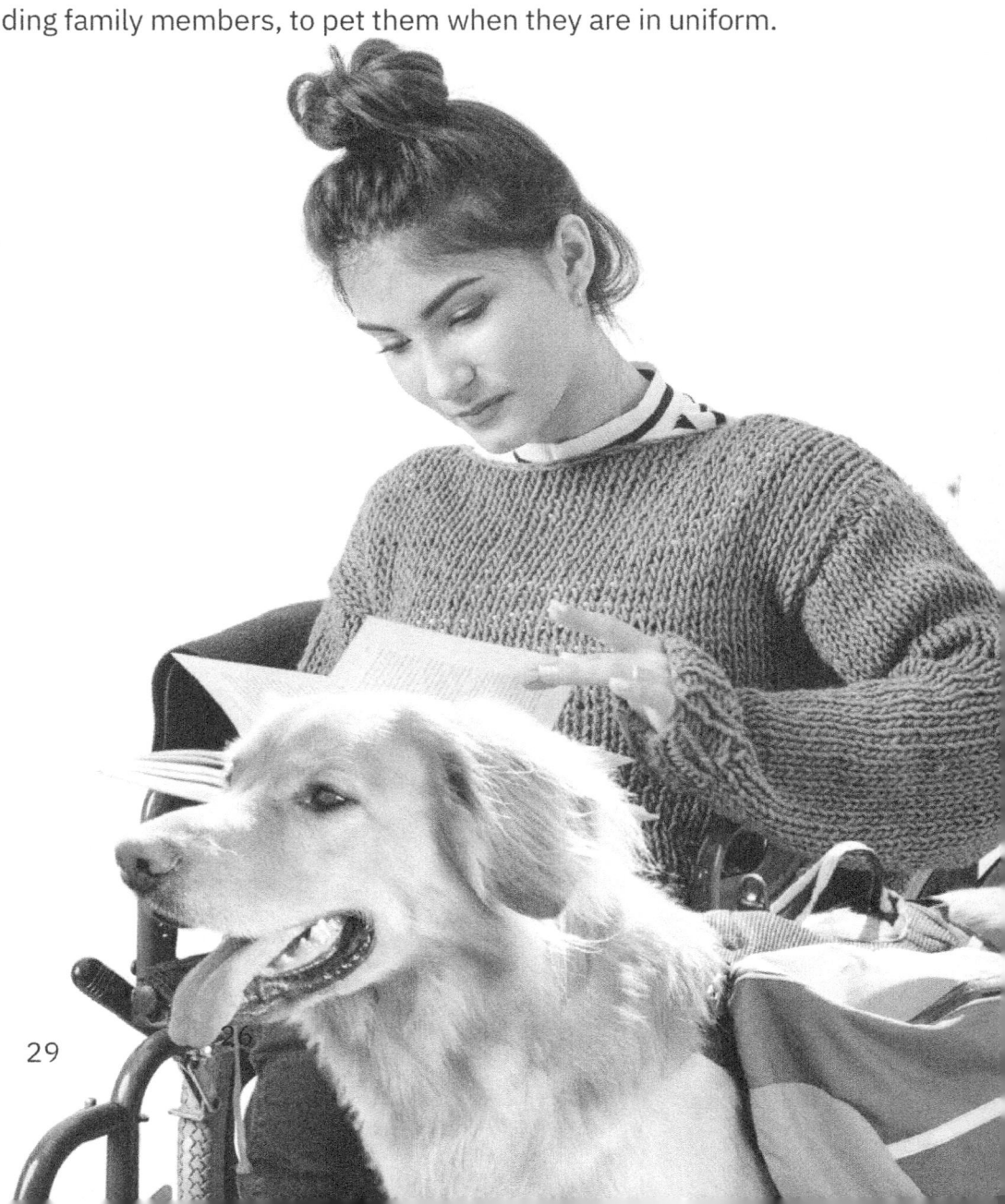

LEASH/TETHER/HARNESS

ADA law requires service dogs to be leashed/tethered or harnessed for public access unless it would cause them not to be able to perform their trained task.

A proper leash may be made from nylon or leather and the most common length is 4 feet or 6 feet. It is a matter of personal preference, but I have found that longer than 4 feet is too long and can easily get tangled in a wheelchair.

Some handlers use an even shorter leash called a traffic lead or tab, which is basically a handle with a clip and only 18" in length.

Many varieties of collars are on the market. All dogs should wear a flat buckle collar with their tags on it, but in public, you will want to make sure that your dog's collar is not making noise.

They sell a product that goes over the tags to keep them from jingling.

Your service dog should be well-trained by the time you begin public access work so attaching the leash to the flat collar should not be an issue.

I use a slip collar made from nylon with dogs I train because during training, a flat collar sits too low on the neck and dogs sometimes pull against them. This does not allow me to communicate any feedback from the other end of the leash and can cause injury to a dog's throat.

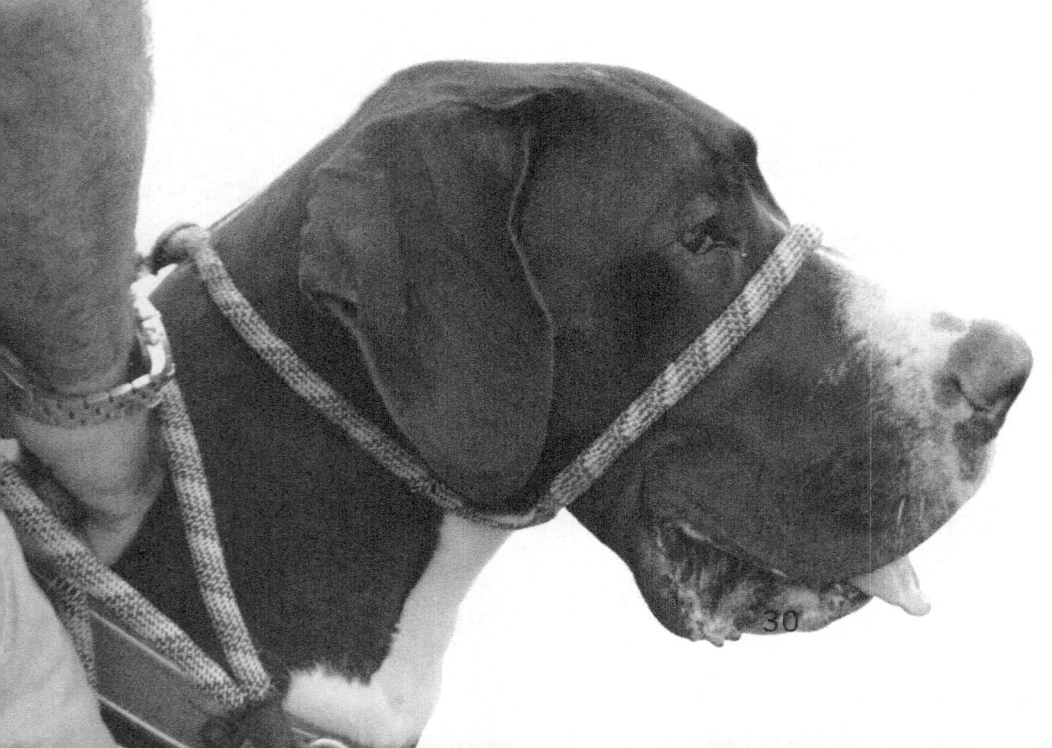

Some dogs do well using a head collar like a gentle leader. Some handlers may also choose to use a head collar because their disability makes it more difficult to train using other types of collars.

It is not against the rules, but I don't believe service dog handlers should use prong collars or metal choke chains.

It is pretty standard across the board that service dogs are trained using reward-based methods only and those types of collars are not used by trainers who only use positive reinforcement. In addition, a service dog may have been trained using a prong collar but once the dog is ready for public access work it should be trained well enough not to need that type of collar any longer.

If your dog still needs a prong collar and will not walk correctly without it, s/he needs more training. I suggest further training be performed without the prong or choke collar for best results.

Harnesses are made for pulling and guiding. The harness puts pressure at the dog's chest, where s/he has the most power to pull into it.

Harnesses should be custom made if they are to be worn full time. Harnesses also should be checked routinely for wear that may cause discomfort from pressure points.

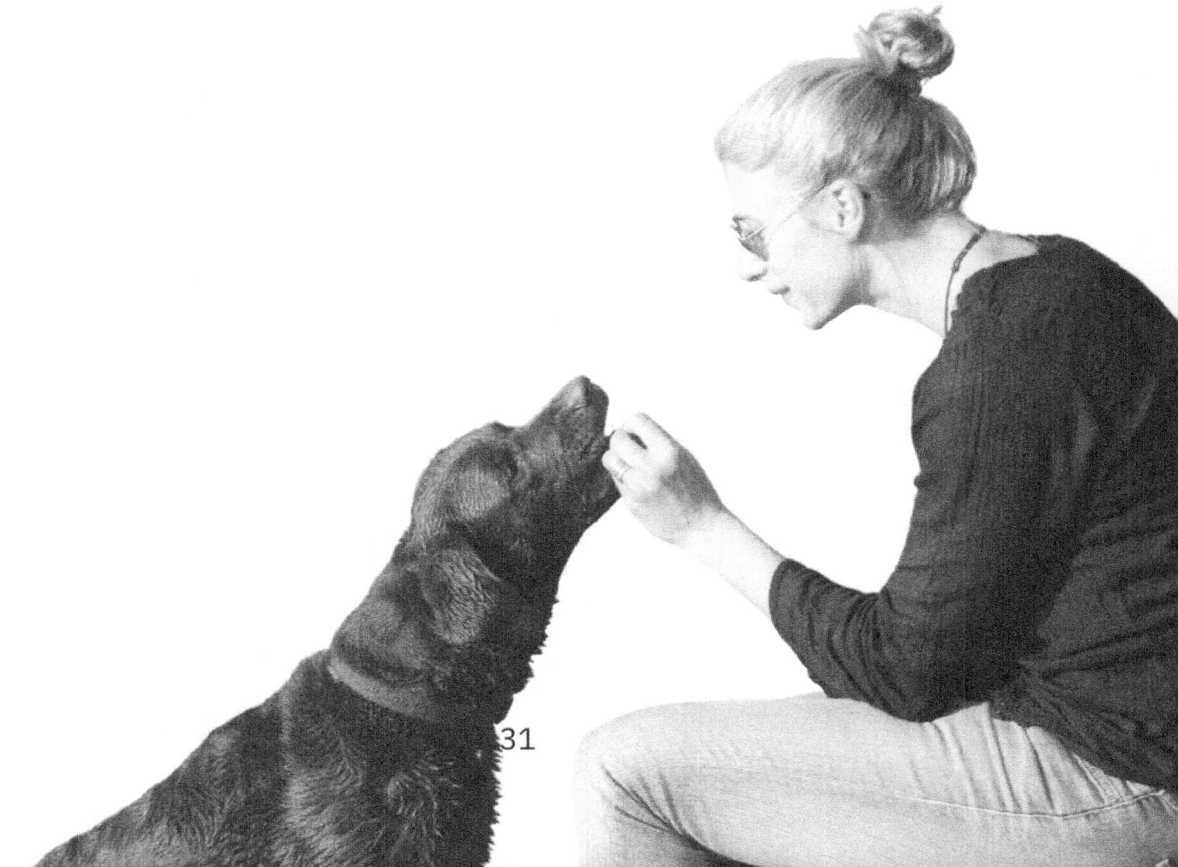

BOOTIES

All service dogs should have well-fitting booties if their work includes having their feet exposed to weather extremes. Summer weather can raise the temperature of asphalt or concrete to the point that your dog's feet suffer serious burns.

The salt used to melt snow in the winter can cause irritation to a service dog's paw pads as well.

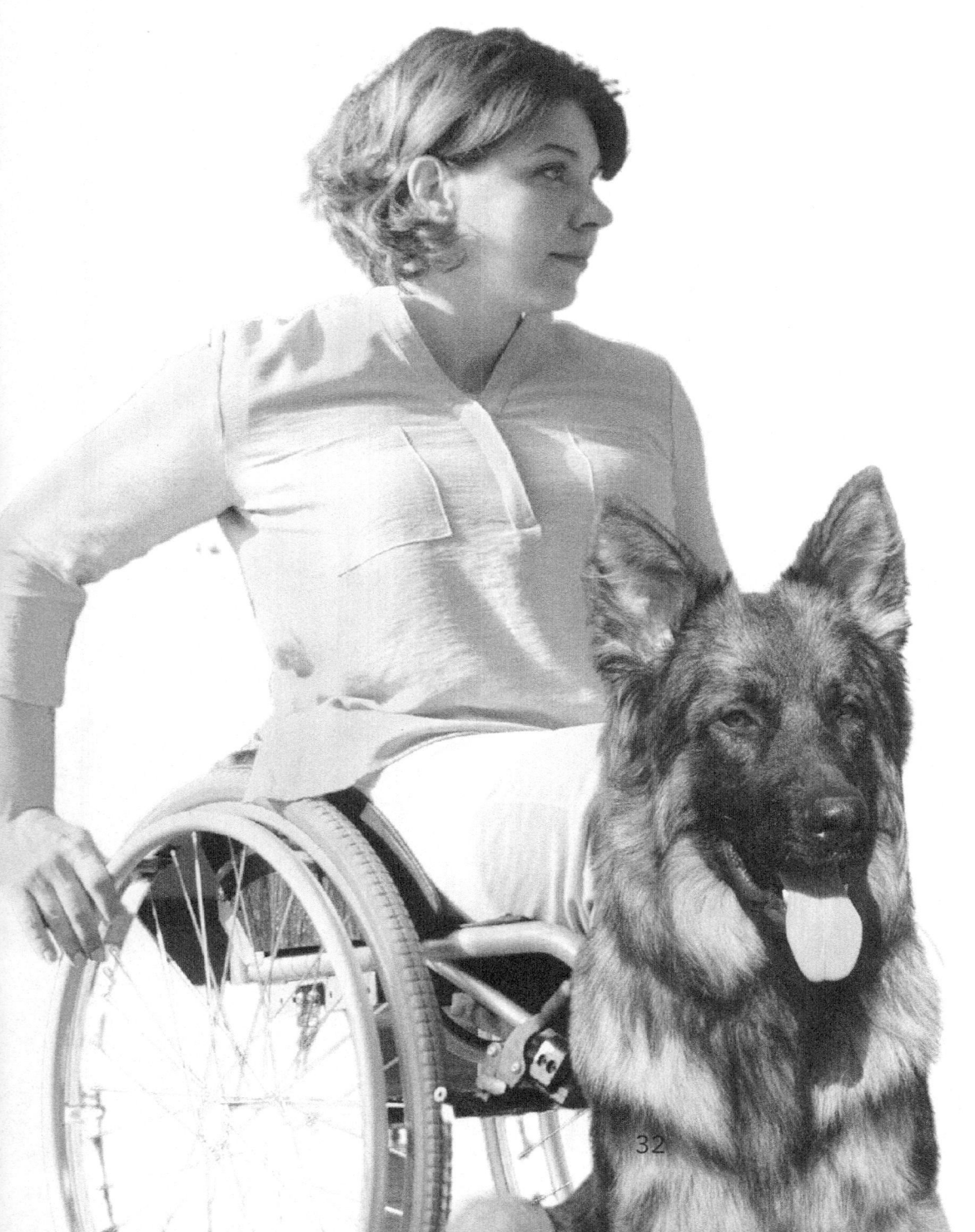

CHAPTER 5:
ARE YOU READY TO BEGIN PUBLIC ACCESS TRAINING?

ESSENTIAL BEHAVIOR

Service dogs must behave a certain way in public. This is important because as a service dog handler you are representing all service dog teams. Service dogs should not be taken into public unless they follow this etiquette.

SERVICE DOGS

• Should be virtually invisible to other people

• Lie out of the way in restaurants and other establishments

• Focus on their handler 100% of the time

• Are quiet

• Ignore other people

• Walk next to their handler (unless the task includes leading or pulling a wheelchair)

• Ignore other service dogs/animals

• Respond to cues given by their handler

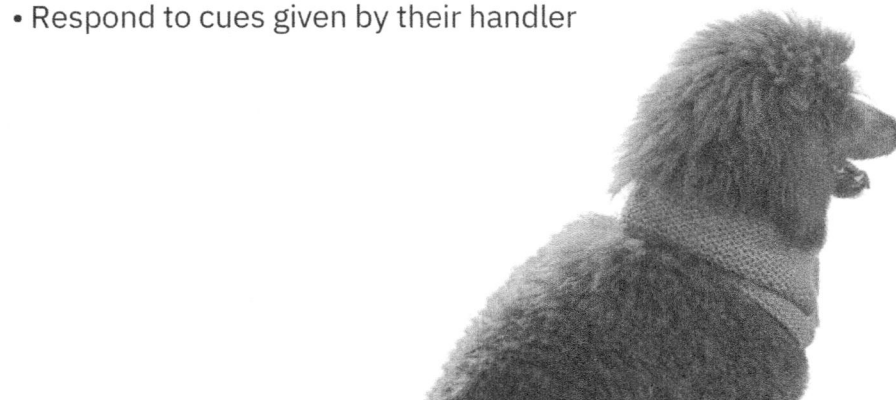

WHILE IN PUBLIC, SERVICE DOGS DO NOT:

• Show aggression of any sort

• Bark or whine (unless part of an alert task)

• Eliminate unless cued to do so in a designated area

• Sniff displays or other people

• Beg at the table or eat food dropped on the floor

• Seek attention from people

• Strain at the leash

• Get distracted by other animals

• Act nervous or afraid

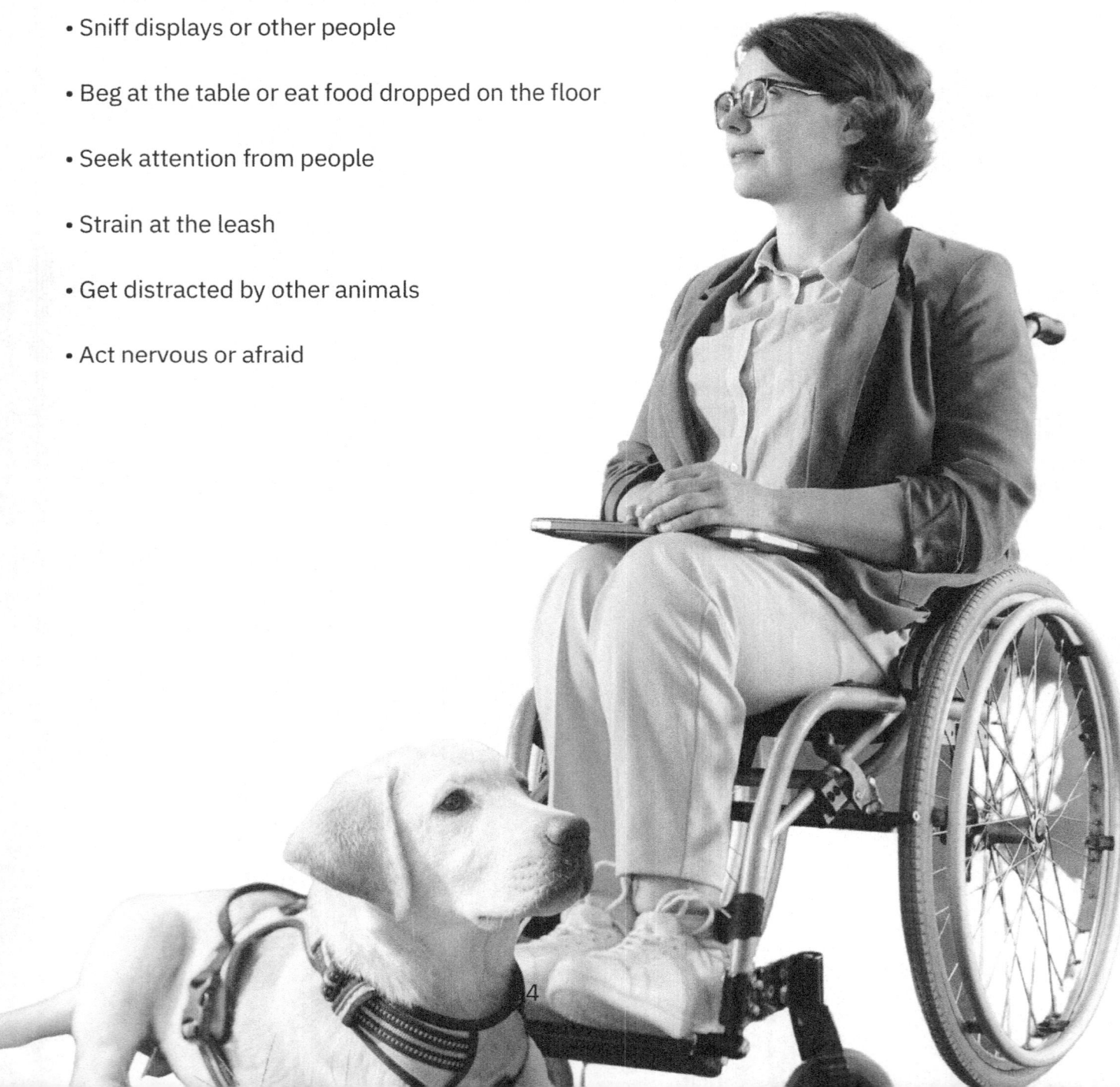

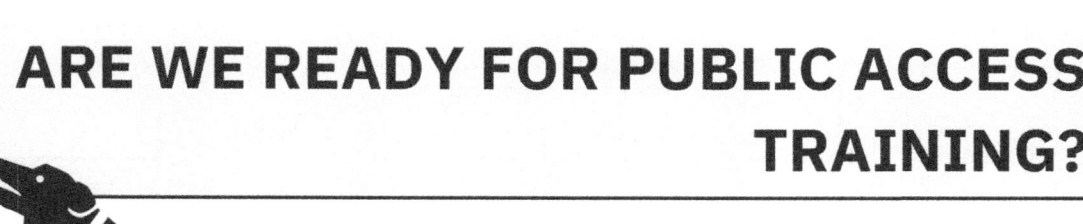

ARE WE READY FOR PUBLIC ACCESS TRAINING?

	ALWAYS	NEEDS WORK
Have you practiced enough that your SDiT can *generalize* skills in any place/situation?		
Is your dog able to ignore people and other animals to focus on you?		
Is your SDiT able to focus on you no matter what distractions are present?		
Have you successfully completed The AKC Canine Good Citizen Program (or similar)?		
Has your SDiT been trained in at least one task to assist with a limitation caused by a disability?		
Is your SDiT housebroken and able to relieve his/herself when given a "cue"?		
Do you understand the legalities when it comes to public access both at a Federal level and your state laws (for example, ADA does NOT cover SDiT's, however, your state may)		
Is your SDiT comfortable in new situations and adjusts right away, without showing nervousness?		

PUBLIC ACCESS READINESS EVALUATION

EVALUATOR: _____   DATE: _____

LOCATION(S): _____

SKILL	DISTRACTIONS	SCORE
Focus on handler		🦴🦴🦴🦴🦴
Advanced heel		🦴🦴🦴🦴🦴
Leave-it		🦴🦴🦴🦴🦴
Down-stay		🦴🦴🦴🦴🦴
Ignore other people		🦴🦴🦴🦴🦴
Controlled reaction to other dogs		🦴🦴🦴🦴🦴
		🦴🦴🦴🦴🦴
		🦴🦴🦴🦴🦴
		🦴🦴🦴🦴🦴
		🦴🦴🦴🦴🦴

REMARKS

TOTAL SCORE: _____

FINAL TEST DATE: _____

CHAPTER 6: PROOFING AND GENERALIZATION

WHAT DOES IT MEAN TO BE PROOFED?

Proofing is solidifying cues that your dog has learned. When your dog responds to a cue at least 90% of the time, you will begin to add distance, duration, and distractions.

Do not make the mistake of adding them at the same time. When you begin to add a distraction, you will go back through all of the steps beginning at phase one of training the cue with one new distraction criteria at a time.

WHAT IS GENERALIZATION?

Generalization is a dog's understanding that the cue or behavior is performed the same whether they are at home, at the park, at night, if you are standing on your head when you give the cue, and so on.

Humans tend to be great at generalizing, but dogs not so much.

You have to teach each behavior, cue, and task reliably in an area with no distractions, and then teach it from the very beginning in new places (including different rooms in your house) and while you are in different positions (sitting, standing, with your back to the dog, from another room, etc).

Do not worry, each time you go back to the beginning with new criteria your dog will go through the steps faster, and eventually, the behavior will be solid enough that your dog will be able to generalize that behavior to other places and circumstances on his/her own.

TRAINING PROCEDURE TIPS

1. **Begin all new behaviors, cues or tasks by training with NO Distractions at all.** I mean, absolutely nothing! A quiet room with no windows would be ideal. Turn off the T.V. and your phone for the session so you can focus on your dog 100%

2. **Break anything you teach down into the tiniest of steps**, and if that is too much break it down even more. I have included a worksheet just for this essential step

3. **At first, mark and reward any interaction with the item** you want them to work with, even a glance

4. **The dog "gets it" when they will perform what you are asking** 8/10 times (80%) according to most trainers. I like to go for 9/10 (90%). When your dog reaches this milestone is when two things happen:

    A. You begin a random schedule of reinforcement. This means that for that particular behavior, the dog no longer earns a reward every single time. The best way to solidify the behavior is to only reward exceptional demonstrations of the behavior.

    B. You move to the next step in the plan you have mapped out. If you have mastered all of the teaching steps, you will move on to proofing each step.

5. **Each proofing strategy you begin will start at the beginning of Phase I/Step 1.** Go back to marking and rewarding continually for a few repetitions (it will go faster each time as your dog learns to generalize the behavior in different places and in the presence of an array of distractions

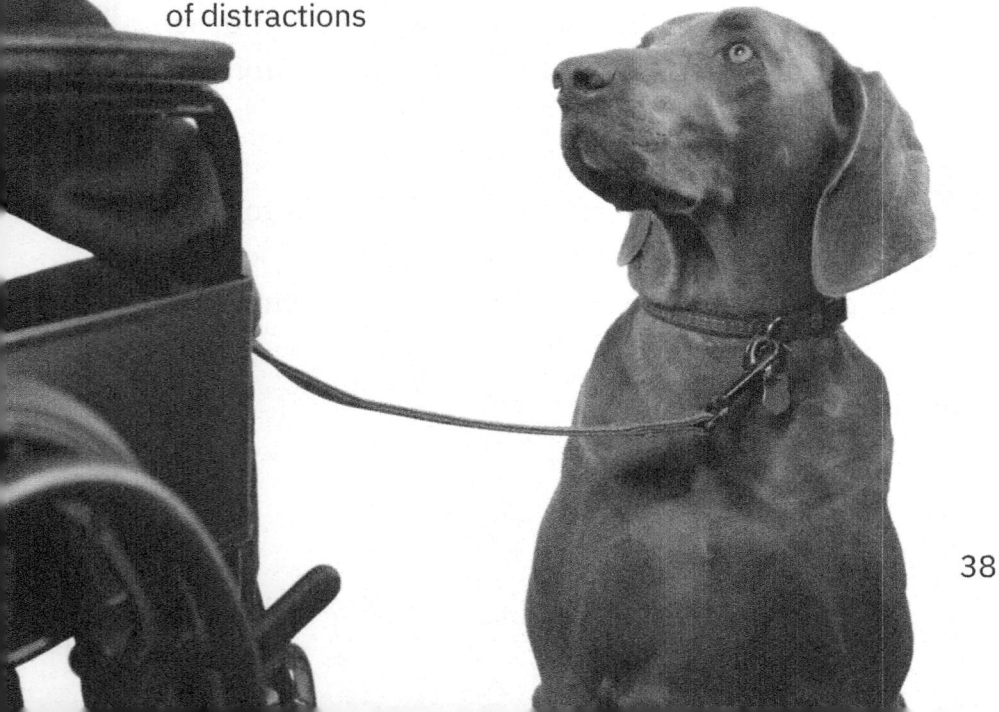

6. **If at any time your dog is having trouble, simply go back a step** or more if necessary. Work at the last step your dog was successful to build confidence and training will become solid

7. **Never EVER get frustrated and yell at or lose patience with your dog** S/he is trying and if you lose your cool, your dog will likely shut down. A dog cannot learn when this happens. If you feel frustrated, STOP the session rather than risk destroying your dog's training. If you find that you lose your patience or become frustrated often, you need to hire a professional trainer to help you

8. **Jackpot *(a handful of food rewards)* milestones** and end each training session while your dog is still interested. Have your dog perform something s/he knows so s/he ends on a success. Further reward the training your dog did with play or something else your dog likes to do, such as a walk

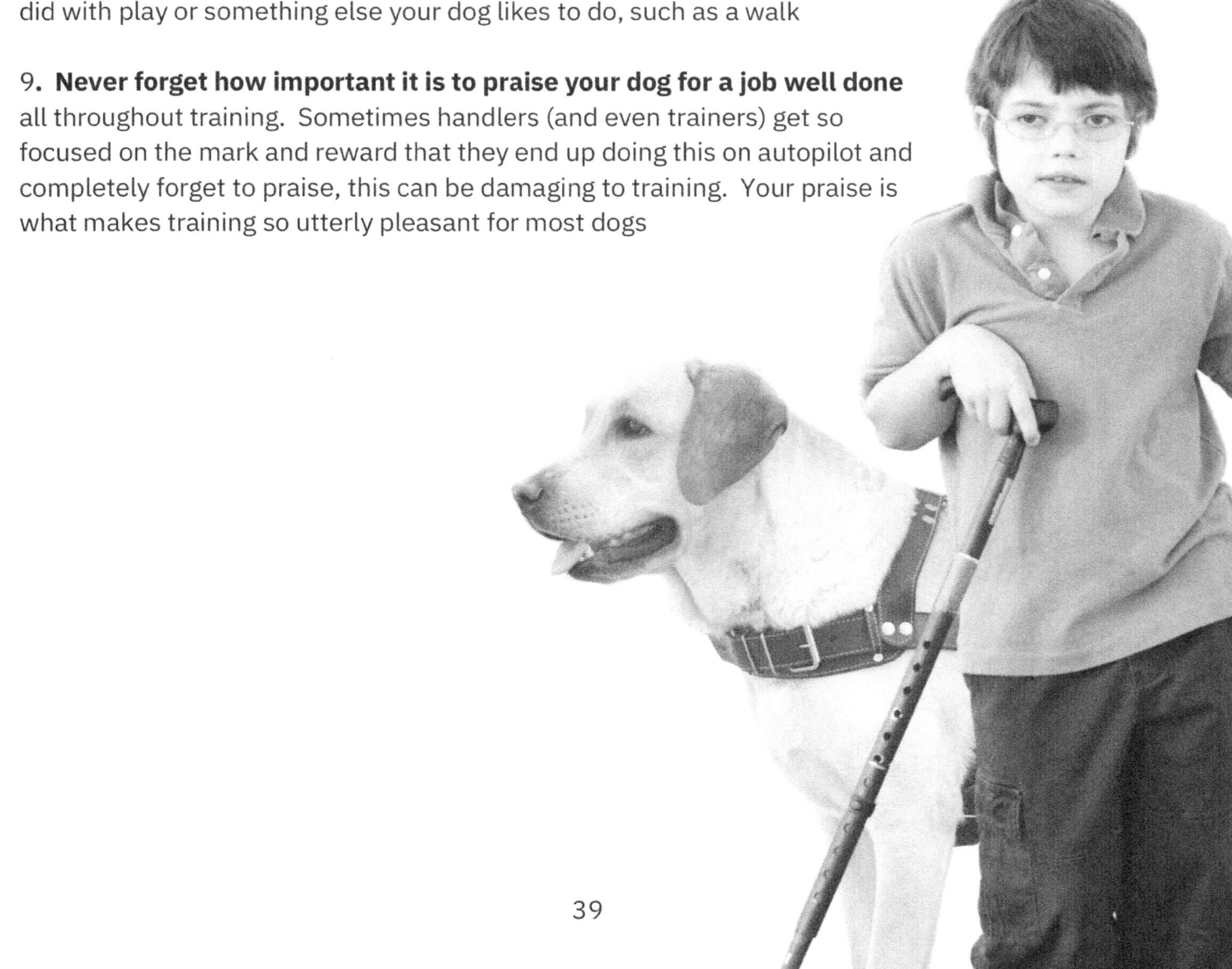

9. **Never forget how important it is to praise your dog for a job well done** all throughout training. Sometimes handlers (and even trainers) get so focused on the mark and reward that they end up doing this on autopilot and completely forget to praise, this can be damaging to training. Your praise is what makes training so utterly pleasant for most dogs

PROOFING WORKSHEET

A behavior is proofed when a dog is able to generalize it to *ANY* place under *ALL* circumstances. Generalizing a behavior means the dog understands that a cue means the same thing at home as it does in the park or if I am in a different position.

For each cue/behavior/task you teach, you will use the examples below to help your dog learn to generaliize. Be creative, come up with your own proofing ideas

For each new behavior you train, practice many repetitions in all situations and gradually add a variety of distractions (one at a time)

DIFFERENT LOCATION
- [ ] IN THE KITCHEN
- [ ] FROM THE DRIVER'S SEAT
- [ ] AT A QUIET PARK
- [ ] THEN AT A BUSY PARK
- [ ] AT THE HARDWARE STORE
- [ ] AT A FRIENDS HOUSE
- [ ]
- [ ]

DIFFERENT DISTANCES
- [ ] 2 FEET AWAY
- [ ] 6 FEET AWAY
- [ ] 22 FEET AWAY
- [ ] FROM THE OTHER ROOM
- [ ] FROM BEHIND A TREE
- [ ] FROM UP IN THE TREE
- [ ] FROM THE TOP OF THE STAIRS
- [ ]

DIFFERENT POSITION
- [ ] CUE GIVEN FACING AWAY FROM DOG
- [ ] CUE FROM SITTING
- [ ] CUE WHILE LAYING DOWN
- [ ] CUE WHILE YOUR DOG IS LAYING DOWN
- [ ] CUE WHILE SITTING ON THE FLOOR
- [ ] WHILE DOING A HANDSTAND
- [ ]
- [ ]

DIFFERENT DISTRACTIONS
- [ ] OTHER ANIMALS 30 FEET
- [ ] KIDS PLAYING 15 FEET
- [ ] WHILE A TRAIN GOES BY 50 FEET
- [ ] CUE WHILE HOLDING AN OPEN UMBRELLA
- [ ] CUE WHILE WEARING A COSTUME
- [ ] CUE IN A WHISPERED VOICE
- [ ]
- [ ]

CHAPTER 7: WATCH FOR SIGNS OF STRESS

Service dogs are constantly exposed to high-stress situations. Even though your service dog has a solid temperament, stress can lead to health issues. It is very important to recognize the signs your service dog may be experiencing stress.

STRESS SIGNALS

- Yawning
- Lip-licking
- Tongue flicking
- Turning head away
- Looking away
- Tail lowering
- Laying ears back
- Breaking eye contact
- Shaking off
- Refusing food
- Ignoring commands
- Heavy panting
- Drooling

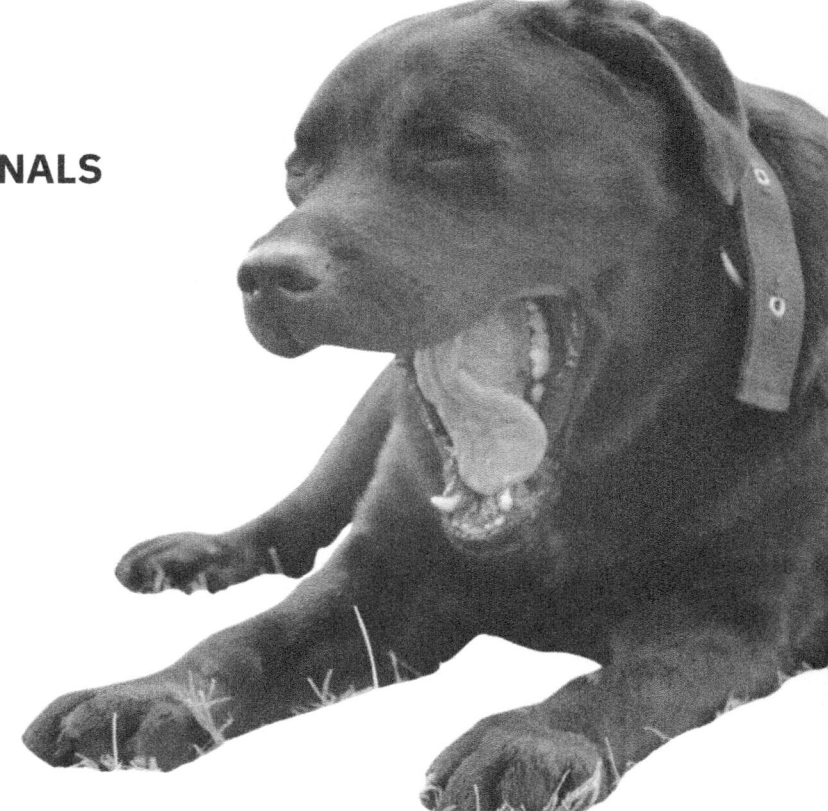

STRESS MANAGEMENT

Many handlers do not realize how stressful of a job it is to be a service dog, even for a dog with a bombproof temperament.

Consider that a service dog may be on call 24 hours a day; spend a great deal of time in places that may be noisy and crowded; their handler may have anxiety or depression; they encounter children and other dogs but must maintain their position; the handler may not be an expert on communication with a dog and misunderstandings can occur; the duties may be physically demanding, and that is just to name a few circumstances that could lead to stress in your service dog.

Stress can lead to health issues and is the leading cause of washing a service dog out from training, and needing to retire them early.

LEARN TO RECOGNIZE SIGNS OF STRESS

It can be difficult for people to read their dog's body language. In fact, most people have a great deal of trouble interpreting canine body language.

Dogs communicate primarily using body language and we so often completely miss subtle cues they give that clearly say "I am uncomfortable".

Look closely at the examples below. What do you see? Do you see signs that these dogs are nervous or uncomfortable?

The subtle cues that dogs give are called calming signals.

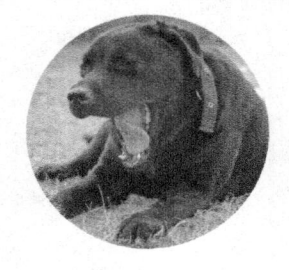

YAWNING
This dog is not sleepy. Yawning is one way that dogs tell you they feel uncomfortable or scared.

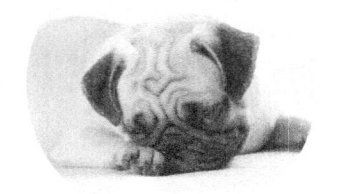

SNIFFING THE GROUND
The "ground sniff" looks casual, and you may not even notice it. However, it is a clear signal that your dog is likely feeling anxious or unsure.

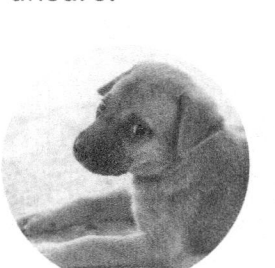

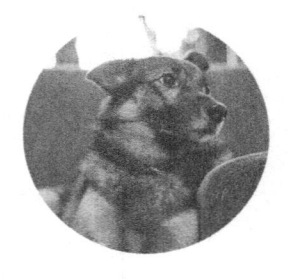

TURNING HEAD AWAY/TO THE SIDE
This is very clear to recognize. A dog feeling stressed that wants to avoid the situation may turn his/her head to the side.

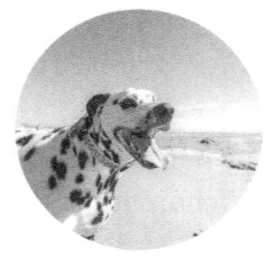

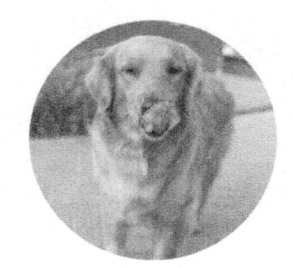

LICKING LIPS
Another clear signal of stress and anxiety is licking of the lips.

HALF-MOON EYES
When a dog looks at you from the side and is showing the whites of his/her eyes, this means they are feeling nervous or unsure as well.

EXTREME PANTING
When a dog is panting with the corners of their lips pulled back all the way, the dog is under extreme stress. A dog in this state will not usually take food.

HOW CAN I HELP PREVENT OR RELIEVE MY SERVICE DOG'S STRESS?

• Use reward-based training (positive reinforcement) when you train your service dog. Avoid using any punishment, losing your patience, or yelling at your dog

• Service dogs need to be able to think independently at times. Punishment and harsh training suppress this by causing a dog to fear to disobey

• Set your dog up for success during training and you will build confidence. End sessions on a positive note with something your dog knows well so you can both celebrate

• Train cues/tasks in small steps and train thoroughly so there is never confusion about whether your dog truly knows what is expected. Train until reliable (90%) and only then add distractions, duration, and distance ONE CRITERIA at a time. When you add a new distraction, ease up on the other expectations
For example, if your dog does a 5-minute sit-stay and you plan to move farther away from them today you would only have them do a 1-minute sit-stay at first
.

• If you have your puppy before the age of 12 or even 16 weeks, ensure that you take extra care to socialize him/her with as many people and situations as you possibly can. The primary socialization window closes at this age and there are no do-overs. Lack of early socialization can destroy the chances a dog has to adjust well enough for service dog work

• Make it a point to teach your dog extensively to be able to "settle"/lie down quietly while in public and add the intensity of distractions and proximity of distance very gradually. If this factor is not given adequate focus, your dog would likely remain on edge when expected to hold a down-stay with what might seem like chaos unfolding around them!

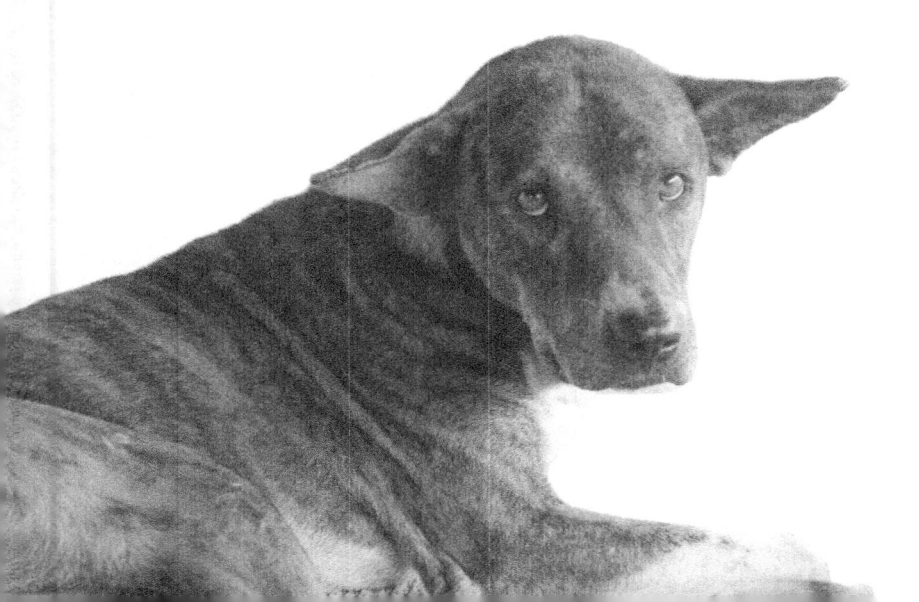

- Learn to recognize stress signals that your dog may be showing. These signs can be misinterpreted for something else like stubbornness or laziness and can be easy to miss completely if you are not fluent in speaking "dog"

- If your dog shows signs of stress during training or in public, stop immediately. Get them out of the situation and change the mood. If it happens on a regular basis or suddenly, contact your trainer right away to prevent permanent damage to your training

- Allow your dog to be a dog sometimes. If your dog likes to play ball or wrestle with the neighbor's dog, ensure you make time for this

- Massage is a great technique for rewarding and relaxing your dog. If you are unable to do it yourself, consider hiring someone or asking a friend/family member to try it

- Your service dog is very tuned in to your well-being. Days, when your condition might be worse physically or emotionally, will affect your dog (whether you notice or not). Keep this in mind on bad days and try to be extra understanding and appreciative of your best friend. After all, their entire life revolves around your needs and we sometimes take this for granted

- Use video both during training and while working in public. Going back and reviewing footage can reveal signs your dog is stressed that you would have otherwise missed and makes it possible to critique your own training habits that could be improved to work better as a team

STRESS EVALUATION

M T W T F S S

LOCATION

MY MOOD

TIME

DATE

PROXIMITY
- ☐ Inside the establishment
- ☐ Outside the establishment

ENVIRONMENT

DURATON
TOTAL MINUTES

TRIGGERING EVENT

STRESS SIGNS PRESENT
- ☐ COWERING
- ☐ PANTING
- ☐ TREMBLING
- ☐ DROOLING
- ☐ REFUSING FOOD
- ☐ LICKING LIPS
- ☐ SNIFFING THE GROUND
- ☐ YAWNING
- ☐ INABILITY TO FOCUS
- ☐ TUCKED TAIL
- ☐ SHAKING OFF
- ☐ AVOIDANCE
- ☐ WHALE EYE
- ☐ GROWLING
- ☐ BITING
- ☐ BARKING
- ☐ OTHER

DESCRIPTION OF INCIDENT

ACTION PLAN
- ☐ GO BACK A STEP
- ☐ CONTACT A PROFESSIONAL
- ☐ DISCONTINUE PUBLIC ACCESS TRAINNG/WASHOUT
- ☐ DESENSITIZE
- ☐ OTHER

STRESS EVALUATION NOTES

CHAPTER 8: HOW TO GET STARTED

PET-FRIENDLY LOCATIONS

Before taking your dog into public places that do not generally allow animals, make sure you do plenty of practice in pet-friendly establishments.

Do not dress your dog in a vest during these outings because socialization is the goal and your dog is not yet working.

If you are raising a young puppy (under 12 weeks), use these outings for as much socialization as you can squeeze in. Allow people to pet your puppy and make it a point to expose your puppy to a variety of stimuli (i.e. shopping carts, noisy crowds, traffic at a safe distance, balloons, children of all ages, etc).

Make sure that all of these experiences are positive ones. If your puppy or dog begins to show any signs of stress, remove them from the situation immediately.

Do not, under any circumstances, force your puppy to endure something that scares him/her. This technique is called "flooding" and can backfire when used on a puppy during the primary socialization window or during a fear impact period. You probably will not even know when your puppy is experiencing a fear-impact period and a scary experience could have devastating permanent effects that would ruin a puppy's future as a service dog.

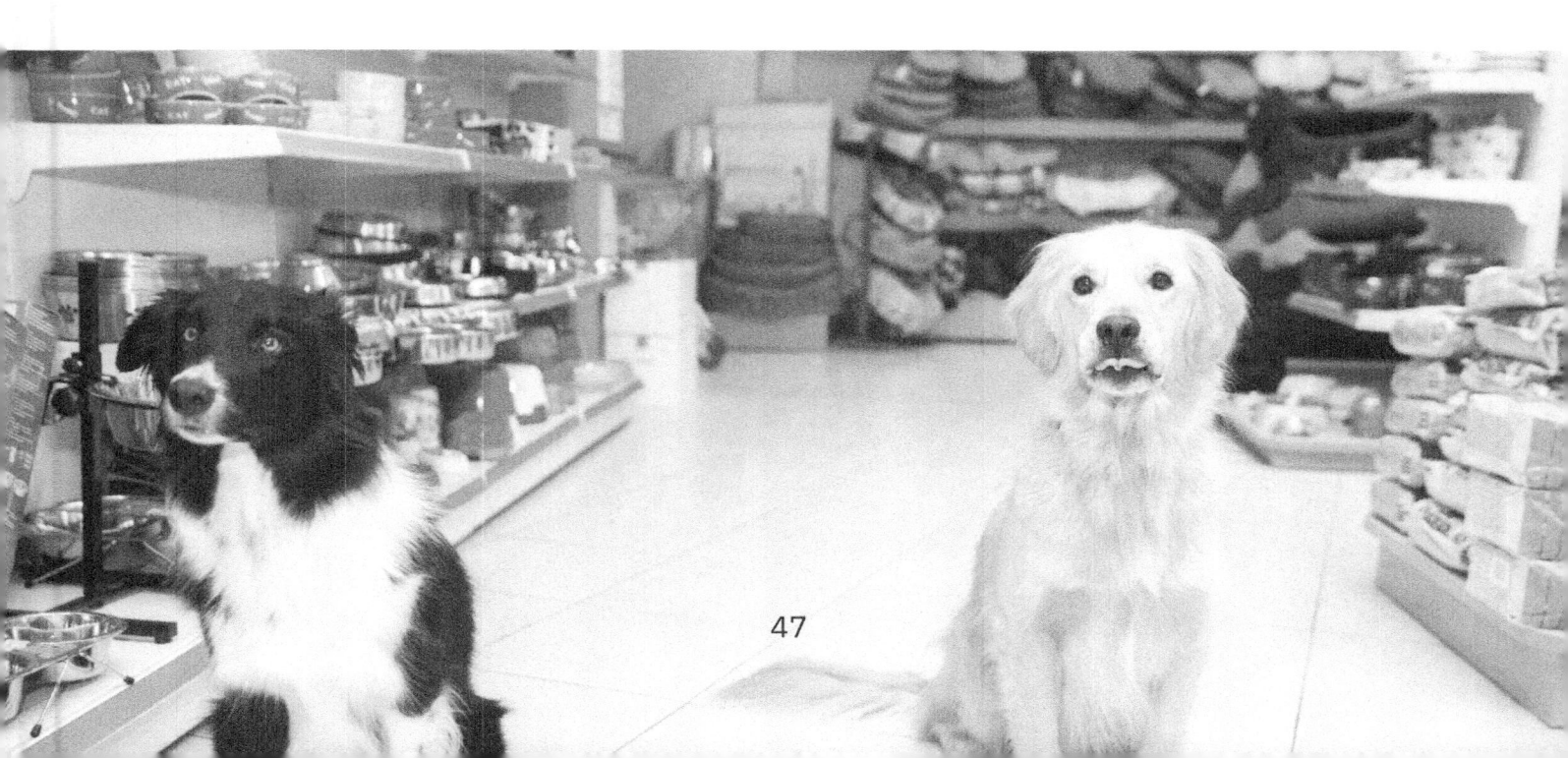

BACK TO PHASE I

When you begin training in public, you cannot expect your dog to jump right in at the same level of training that you have been doing at home.

Instead, it is very important to go back to the beginning as if your dog has never been taught in each new place and each new situation. Training will go much faster this time, but you must ensure your dog understands that a cue means the same thing whether you are at home, in a restaurant or boarding an airplane.

To ensure that your dog is comfortable enough and to avoid the possibility of ruining your dog's public access career by moving too fast, you will start slow and begin training outside a building you plan to practice in.

Practice cues in the parking lot on off-peak hours when it is likely to be less busy. When your dog is comfortable and performs all cues asked 95% of the time, move closer to the building and start from the beginning there.

Then practice in the parking lot when it is busy. Move onto the front of the building when it is busy.

When you do finally enter the establishment, make sure you go on a day and time when it is not busy.

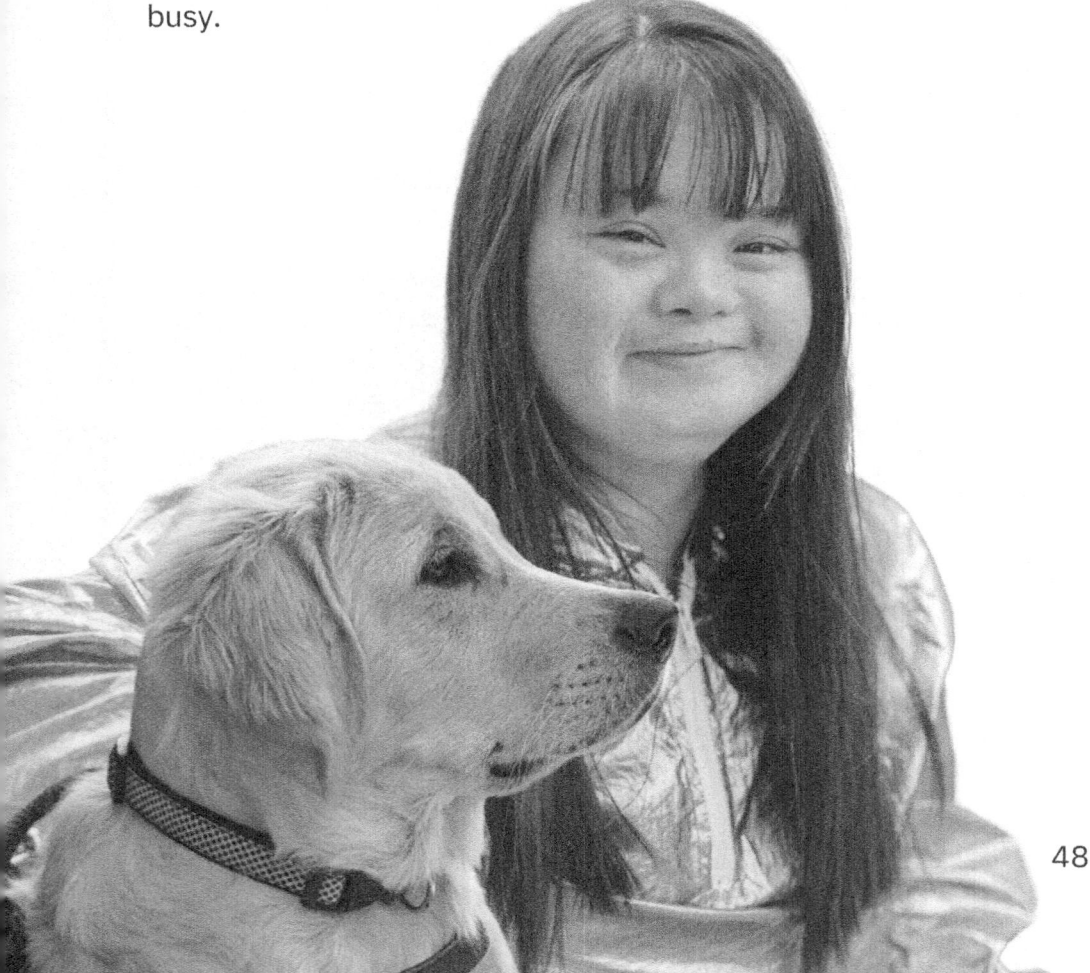

FIRST PUBLIC ACCESS OUTINGS

Follow this example for gradually acclimating your dog to public places. Perform each step until your dog is comfortable and able to focus on you only. Do not be afraid to go back a step if your dog has trouble.

If your dog shows signs of stress, stop immediately and resume training in a place and distance where your dog is comfortable.

01 Practice cues outside of the establishment

02 Enter and immediately exit the establishment

03 Enter and take a brief stroll through the store and then exit

04 Enter and practice a few sits and downs, then exit

05 Enter and purchase one item, then exit

06 Begin from step 1 in a new establishment

YOUR MARKERS

Duration Marker

I use the clicker or "Yes!"

This marker is used when your dog is expected to continue performing the cue s/he was given.

For example, you ask your dog to down. Your dog is expected to stay in a down until released using either a release word or the termination marker in early training.

Termination Marker

I use "Free!"

This marker is used when want your dog to terminate the behavior you had asked them to continue and come to you for a reward.

For example, you want to release your dog from the platform. When you say the termination marker, your dog should get off the platform and come to you for the reward.

No-reward Marker

I use "Nope!"

This marker is used when want your dog makes a mistake. It is given calmly and is NOT a correction.

For example, your dog is on the platform and gets off without being released. Within one second of breaking, you give the no-reward marker and calmly use the leash to lead the dog back to the platform.

CHAPTER 9: ESSENTIAL TESTS

AKC CANINE GOOD CITIZEN AND BEYOND

THE CANINE GOOD CITIZEN PROGRAM

The American Kennel Club (AKC) has several programs geared at encouraging well-behaved dogs.

The first is the S.T.A.R. Puppy, an incentive program that encourages responsible puppy ownership during a 6-week class taught by an AKC Canine Good Citizen Evaluator.

There are 20 test items, some of which grade you on responsible acts such as bringing poop bags to class ad having an ID tag on your puppy. Other test items evaluate social skills and prepare puppies to take the Canine Good Citizen Exam in the future.

I highly recommend that anyone raising a service dog from a puppy enroll in a S.T.A.R. Puppy class. They are easy to find with CGC evaluators virtually everywhere and very affordable. After S.T.A.R. Puppy, you can get your Canine Good Citizen Certification. The CGC is pretty simple but teaches great skills to prepare for public access, especially working around other dogs.

Dogs that are registered purebreds by the AKC earn a title when they pass the CGC.

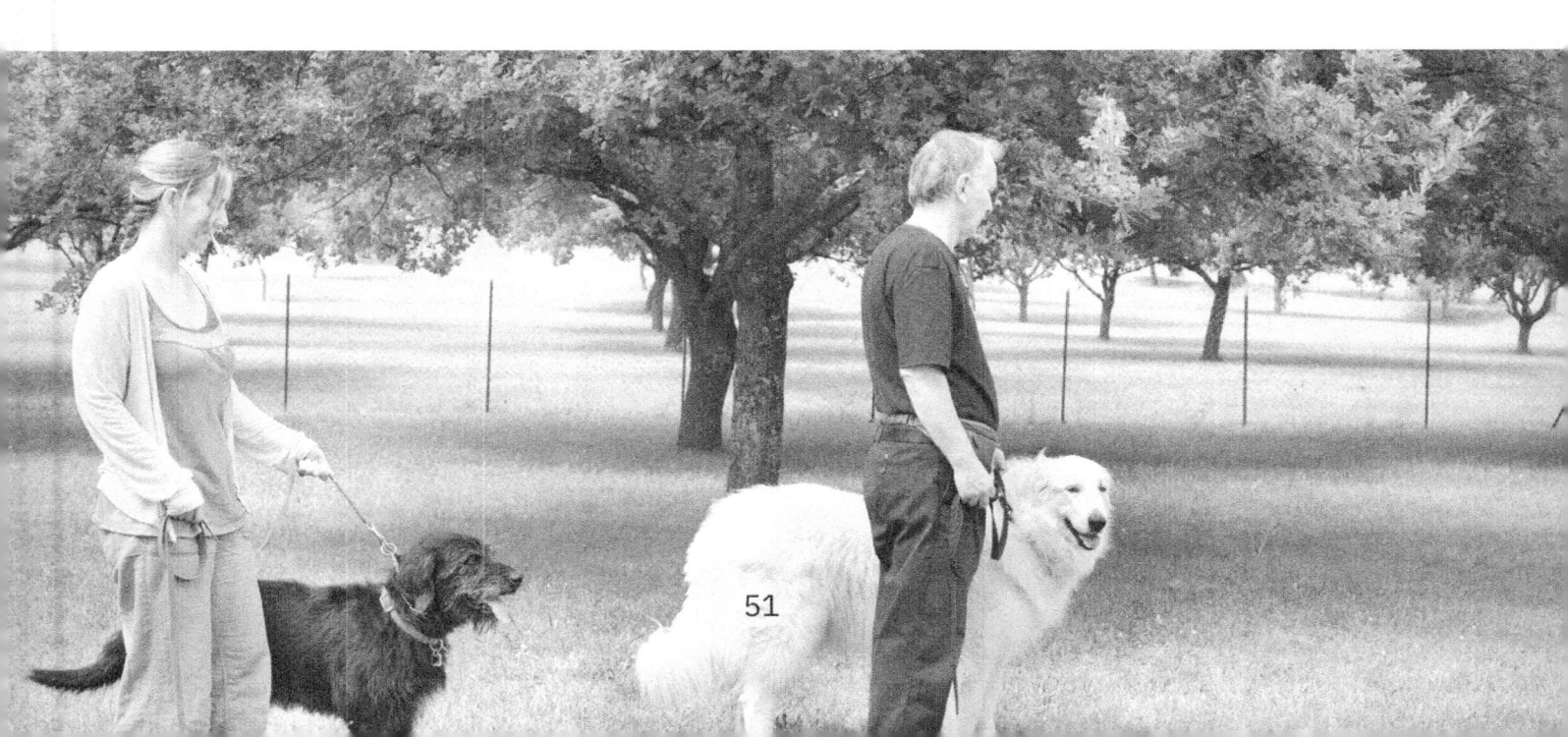

BEYOND THE CGC

The AKC has added several new programs to the CGC family dog program. After you pass the CGC, especially if your state is one that does not permit your SDiT to train in public, you would be wise to take advantage of the widely spread and inexpensive testing options.

After the CGC if you want to take the next step your dog will need to be AKC registered if they are not already. Dogs that are purebred but not eligible for AKC registration will get a PAL (purebred alternative listed) number. Mixed breeds need a Canine Partners number to participate in the next programs.

These registration numbers cost a one-time fee which is relatively inexpensive. It is definitely worth it.

Once your dog has an AKC number, you can participate in the Advanced CGC; Community Canine (CGCA).

The last test in the CGC family dog program is the CGC Urban Canine, which the AKC refers to as a "Public Access Test" but not necessarily for service dog work.

If you still have time after all four of these certifications, the AKC has a therapy dog program, a trick dog program, and multiple sports programs.

The AKC also recently released a scent work program as well as The AKC Temperament Test. I do not receive a commission in any way for promoting these AKC activities; I promote them because I truly believe in it for service dog trainees.

The truth is, I have actually been an AKC Canine Good Citizen Evaluator for 14 years and just recently after they released the Temperament Test I took a course and a test in order to ensure I was experienced enough to become a Temperament Test Evaluator.

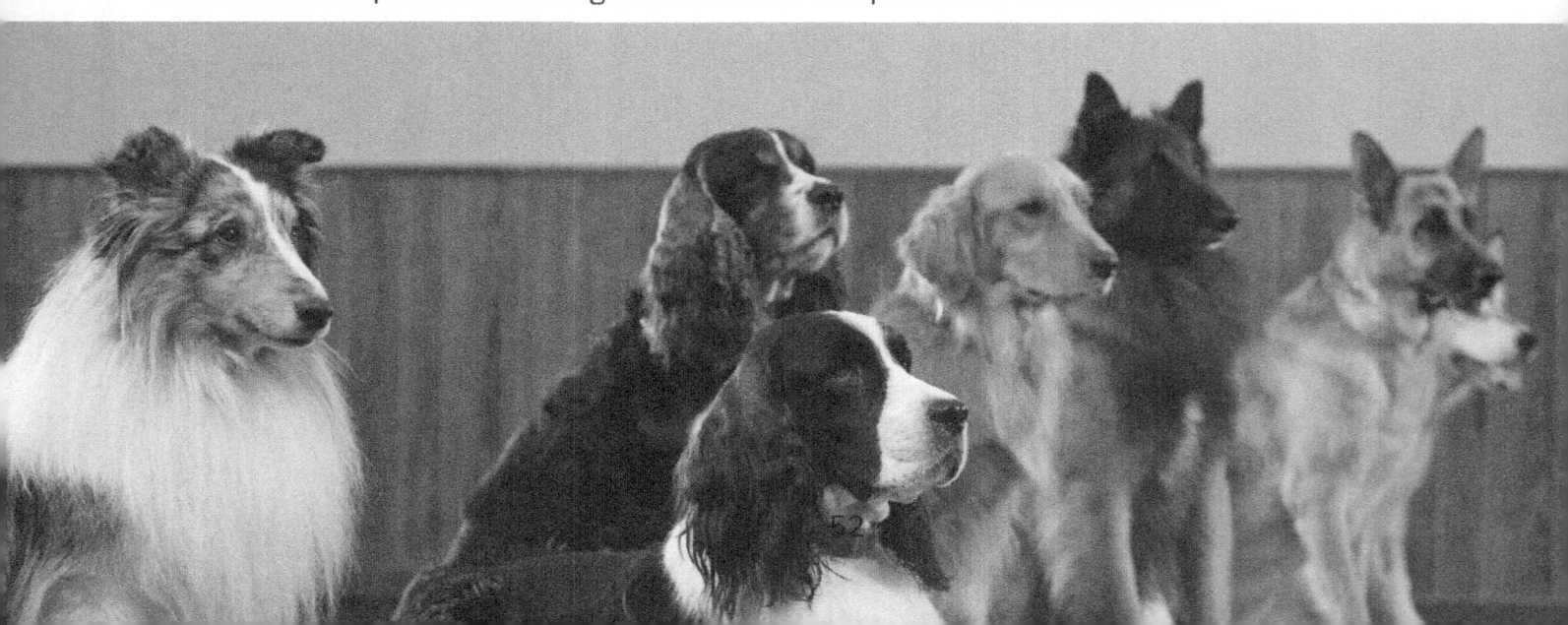

ADI PUBLIC ACCESS TEST

Assistance Dogs International (ADI) is an organization that has developed some standards for minimum training requirements a service dog should have before public access. Overall, the service dog community accepts the guidelines the ADI has suggested.

The first Public Access Test that I know of was created by the ADI, and service dog trainers and owner trainers have used their test for public access training since the beginning.

The ADI decided recently that their test should not be used unless the tester is ADI accredited.
The ADI is a reputable organization and if your trainer or program is accredited by the ADI, you can be certain that you are in good hands. Unfortunately for many skilled trainers, ADI accrediting is geared toward large non-profits.

Smaller organizations, ones that are just starting, and individual trainers would have a difficult time meeting the criteria for ADI accreditation. This means that suddenly many service dog trainers were asked not to utilize the ADI test any longer.

No problem! There are now several public access tests that are free for anyone to use. In fact, most of these other tests are more in-depth than the ADI test.

TASK FOUNDATION TRAINING

PASS

"Pass" is similar to the "Swing Finish", except that the dog follows your right index finger to come from the front position (facing you), along your right side and behind your back to finish by sitting on your left side (facing forward) in the "Heel" position.

This can also be the foundation for training a "Got your 6" cue for demanding people give you space in crowded places.

★1 With your dog on leash in the "Front" position; place a treat between your thumb and second finger on your right hand. Put your index finger up for the hand signal

★2 Put your hand, with the treat in front of your dog's nose. Extend your arm out to your side as you see in the photo and slowly lead your dog using the lure to go along your right side

★3 If possible, pass the treat behind your back or have another treat you can put in your other hand (still luring the dog) so s/he goes behind you and finishes by coming to your left side and faces forward beside you

★4 Cue "Sit"

★5 Mark and reward

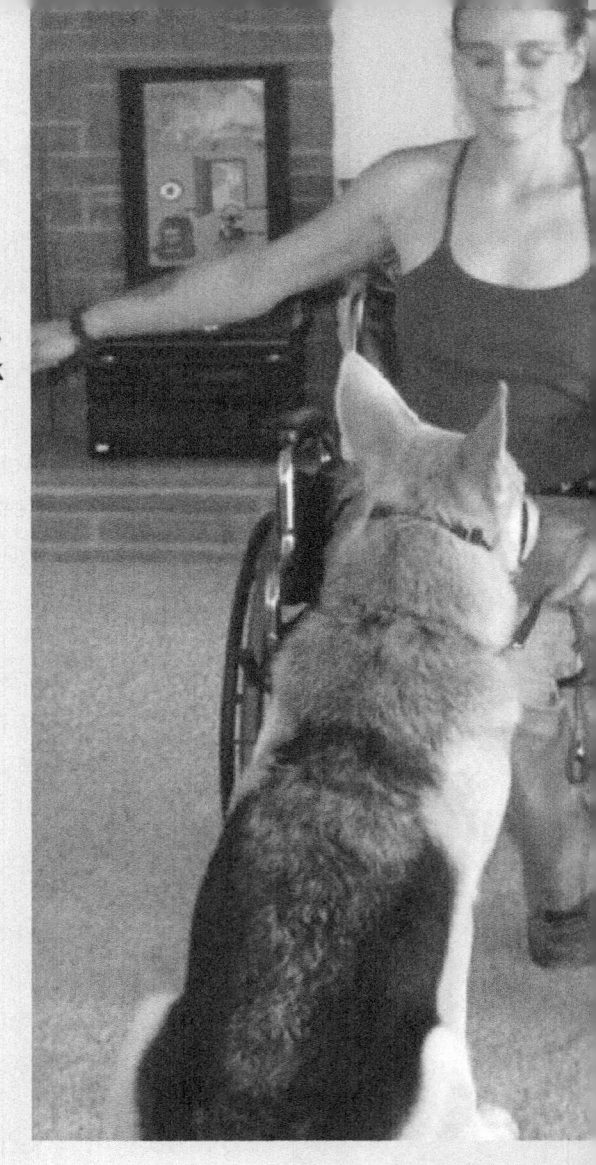

PUBLIC ACCESS

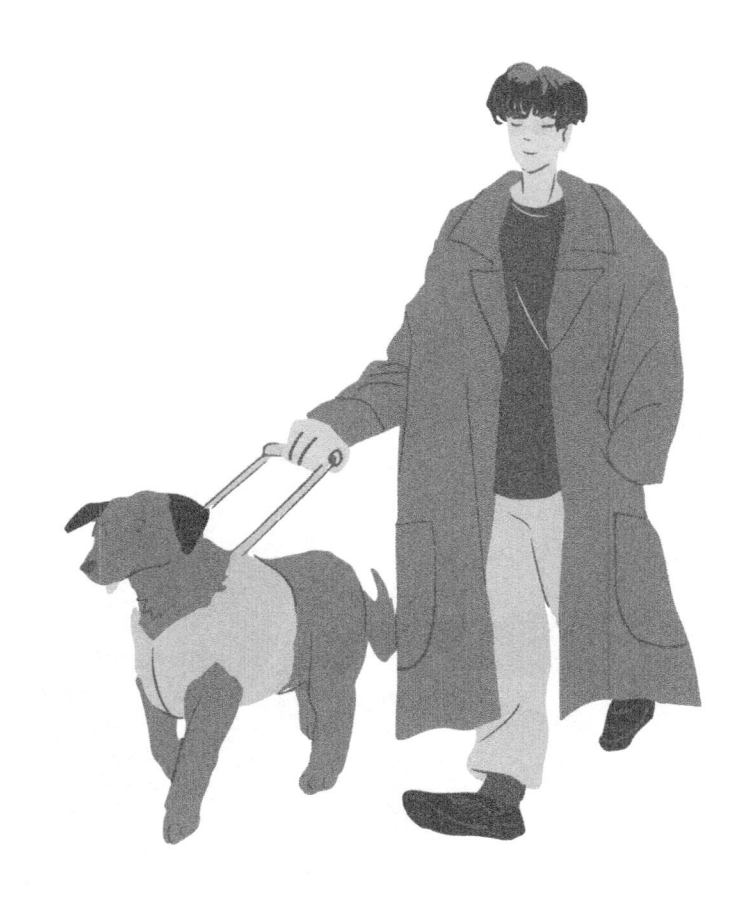

PRACTICE TEST

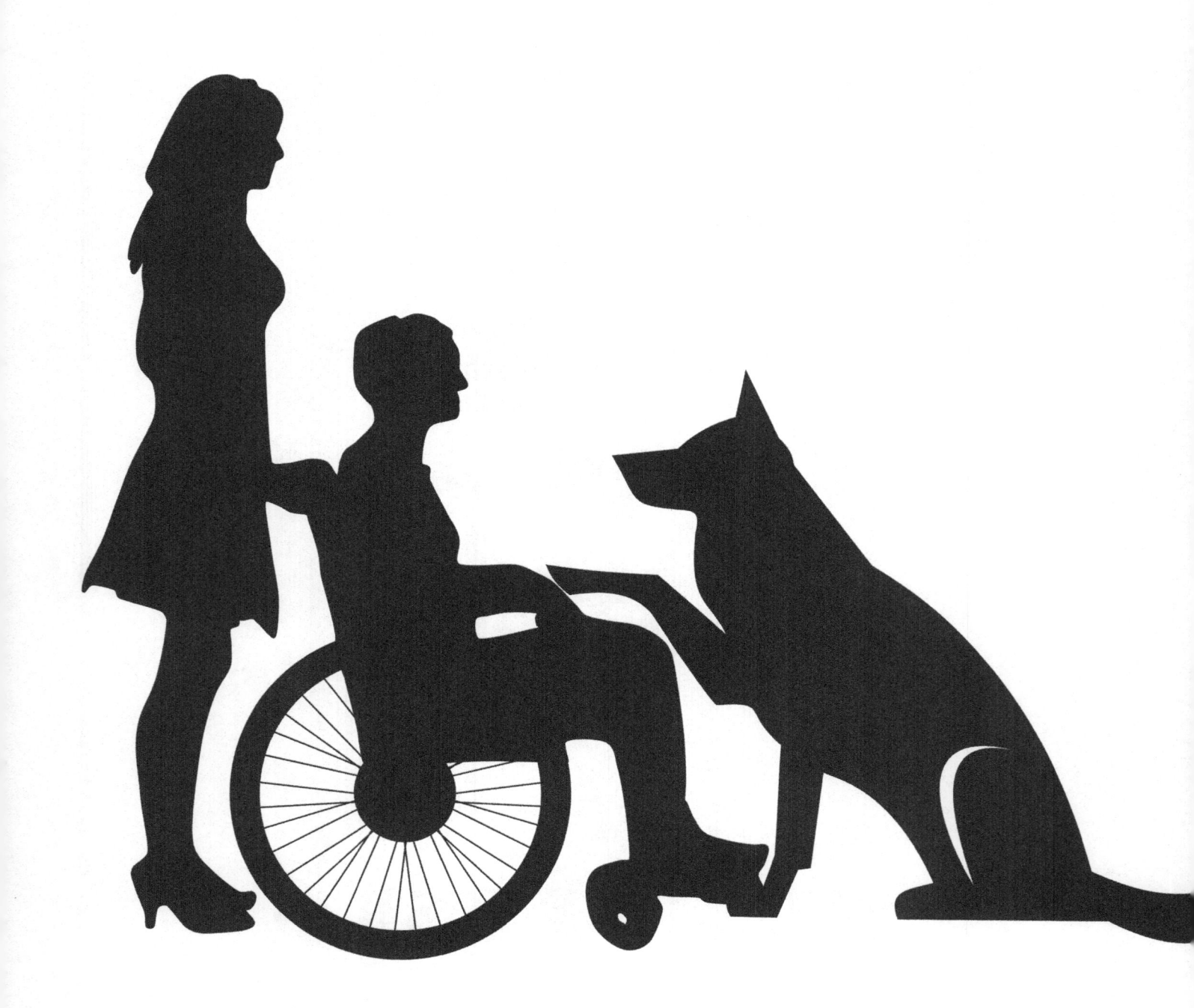

PUBLIC ACCESS EXAM

1) DOG WAITS FOR PERMISSION TO LOAD, ENTERS VEHICLE WHEN CUED BY HANDLER

- The examination begins when handler and service dog-in-training enter the vehicle
- This may be a passenger vehicle or public transportation such as a taxi or city bus
- The dog should wait to be given a cue to enter the vehicle and load without issues
- Handlers should ensure the safety of the dog by use of a crate or other safety device such as a restraint system inside the vehicle when appropriate

2) DOG APPEARS RELAXED WHILE IN VEHICLE/PUBLIC TRANSPORTATION

- The dog should be relaxed and not exhibit anxiety or nervous behavior

3) DOG WAITS IN VEHICLE UNTIL RELEASED

- The dog waits calmly until handler releases him/her from the vehicle
- The dog exits the vehicle in an orderly manner and either sits, stands, or lies down as the handler grabs personal items and secures the vehicle

4) DOG SHOWS APPROPRIATE REACTION TO ANOTHER DOG.

- This portion can be completed at any time during the examination
- A neutral dog will be walked across the path of the dog being tested at a distance of 15 feet and handler will cue the dog's attention back to them if necessary
- The testing dog may show mild interest but be able respond to the cue to focus on the handler
- Testing dogs should not get overly excited, vocalize or intensely stare the other dog down

5) DOG REMAINS UNDER HANDLER CONTROL WHEN THE LEASH IS "ACCIDENTALLY" DROPPED.

- This portion can be completed at any time during the examination
- Use discretion as to the safety of the dog (i.e near a busy street)
- Handler drops the leash and stops. The dog should also stop or return to the handler right away if there is distance between them
- Handler may call the dog if necessary but the dog should respond immediately

6) DOG REMAINS IN CORRECT POSITION AS TEAM ENTERS THE ESTABLISHMENT

- The dog should be beside the handler or within a reasonable distance as appropriate for their task
- Dogs should not strain on the leash
- Forward momentum using a proper mobility harness or guide work in harness are examples where a dog is required to work in front of the handler
- Dogs should not display nervousness upon approaching or entering the building

7) DOG AND HANDLER CAN MANEUVER STAIRS OR ELEVATOR

- Handlers can choose which option
- Escalators are discouraged for safety reasons

8) TEAM HAS A SEAT AT A FOOD ESTABLISHMENT, DOG GOES UNDER SEAT/ TABLE OR OTHERWISE POSITIONS ITSELF OUT OF THE WAY

- Handler is able to cue dog to position itself in a manner that does not obstruct walkways

9) DOG SHOWS APPROPRIATE RESPONSE WHEN FOOD IS DROPPED

- At some point during the meal, handler or evaluator will drop food on the floor near the dog
- Handler may use a "leave it" cue if necessary
- Dog should not get up to get the food and if the dog does go for the food item, the dog should respond to one reminder to "leave it"

10) DOG IGNORES PATRONS WHO ATTEMPT TO DISTRACT THEM

- A person unknown to the dog can be recruited or the scenario could happen naturally
- The person or people should try to get the dog's attention (talking to the dog, making kissy noises, etc.)
- The person remains at least 5 feet away
- The dog should not break position and the handler should be able to cue the dog's focus back to them if necessary

11) DOG REMAINS QUIET AND IN PLACE DURING MEAL

- Dog relaxes during the entire time the handler is at the establishment and does not repeatedly get up to reposition
- Dog should not solicit attention from employees or customers
- Dog remains on a down-stay or position handler instructed until released (15-30 min)

12) DOG REMAINS FOCUSED AND IN CORRECT POSITION THROUGHOUT ESTABLISHMENT WITHOUT SNIFFING DISPLAYS OR OTHER PEOPLE

- Team will go through an establishment with a reasonable amount of other people
- The dog should not sniff other people or displays
- Dog should maintain focus on handler
- Dog should appear comfortable and not display signs of stress

13) DOG SHOWS APPROPRIATE RESPONSE TO VISUAL AND NOISE DISTRACTION

- An unexpected noise (metal item dropping, loud horn or airbrakes) AND A visual distraction (umbrella opening, trash bag being filled with air) will be created or could happen naturally
- Dog may startle initially but should recover within 3-5 seconds
- Noise distraction is presented no closer than 10 feet
- Visual and noise distraction may also be combined (metal trash can being knocked over, noisy shopping cart being pushed nearby)
- In the case of combining visual and noise distractions, 2 should be done at different times
- If the dog responds with extreme stress, the examination will terminate

14) HANDLER IS IN CONTROL WHEN EXITING THE BUILDING

- When the team exits the building, the dog should be beside the handler or within reasonable distance as appropriate for their task
- Dogs should not strain at the leash
- The dog is focused on handler and not overly eager to exit the establishment

15) DOG IS CLEAN AND WELL-GROOMED

- The dog appears clean with no unpleasant smell
- Appears to be reasonably groomed
- Nails are acceptable length

16) SAFETY IS OBSERVED BY SECURING DOG IN A CANINE SEATBELT OR CRATE IN THE VEHICLE

- Evaluator confirmation of appropriate safety measures while dog is in the vehicle

17) HANDLER IS PREPARED FOR POTENTIAL ACCESS CHALLENGES

- Evaluator will make sure that the handler is aware of his/her rights and responsibilities
- Handler knows what s/he can be asked by law and what is illegal for businesses to ask
- Handler has an idea of how they would handle a situation where they were denied access or asked to provide "paperwork"
- Tip: Extra credit for carrying ADA law cards that state the law and/or handler rights

18) HANDLER DEMONSTRATES PROPER USE OF GEAR AND/OR TRAINING AIDS

- Evaluator observes that the handler uses any equipment, gear or training aids safely and humanely
- All items fit well and do not cause discomfort
- Equipment is used correctly

19) OVERALL, DOG FOCUSES ON/RESPONDS TO HANDLER

- Evaluator observes that the dog is focused on the handler most of the time
- Evaluator observes that handler is able to get the dog's attention if the dog becomes distracted

20) HANDLER IS PREPARED WITH SUPPLIES FOR DOG WASTE

- This portion will receive all possible points simply for being prepared with supplies to pick up and dispose of waste

PUBLIC ACCESS PRACTICE EXAM

Date:

Handler:

Dog's Name:

Evaluator:

Location:

Part I

1. Dog waits for permission to load, enters vehicle when cued by handler

　　　No　　　　　Yes　　　　　Needs some work

2. Dog appears relaxed while in vehicle/public transportation

　　　No　　　　　Yes　　　　　Needs some work

3. Dog waits in vehicle until released

☐ No ☐ Yes ☐ Needs some work

4. Dog shows appropriate reaction to another dog

☐ No ☐ Yes ☐ Needs some work

5. Dog remains under handler control when the leash is accidentally dropped

☐ No ☐ Yes ☐ Needs some work

Part II

6. Dog remains in correct position as team enters the establishment

☐ No ☐ Yes ☐ Needs some work

7. Dog and handler can maneuver stairs or elevator

☐ No ☐ Yes ☐ Needs some work

8. Team has a seat at a food establishment, dog goes under seat/table. or otherwise positions itself out of the way

☐ No ☐ Yes ☐ Needs some work

9. Dog shows appropriate response when food is dropped

☐ No   ☐ Yes   ☐ Needs some work

10. Dog ignores patrons who attempt to distract them

☐ No   ☐ Yes   ☐ Needs some work

11. Dog remains quiet and in place during meal

☐ No   ☐ Yes   ☐ Needs some work

12. Dog remains focused and in correct position throughout establishment without sniffing displays or other people

☐ No   ☐ Yes   ☐ Needs some work

13. Dog shows appropriate response to visual and noise distraction

☐ No   ☐ Yes   ☐ Needs some work

14. Handler is in control when exiting the building

☐ No   ☐ Yes   ☐ Needs some work

Part III

15. Dog is clean and well-groomed

☐ No   ☐ Yes   ☐ Needs some work

16. Safety is observed by securing dog in a canine seatbelt or crate in the vehicle

☐ No   ☐ Yes

17. Handler is prepared for potential access challenges

☐ No   ☐ Yes   ☐ Needs some work

18. Handler demonstrates proper use of gear and/or training aids

☐ No   ☐ Yes   ☐ Needs some work

19. Overall, dog focuses on/responds to handler

☐ No   ☐ Yes   ☐ Needs some work

20. Handler is prepared with supplies for dog waste

☐ No   ☐ Yes

CHAPTER 10: CHALLENGES

ACCESS CHALLENGES

Although you will encounter employees (gatekeepers) who ask you inappropriate questions, there are only two (2) that you need to answer:

1) Is that a service dog required because of a disability?

and

2) What task(s) is it trained to perform?

That is it. People may word the questions in different ways, but you are not required to provide anyone with more information than that.

EMPLOYEES OF BUSINESSES SHOULD NOT (BUT OFTEN DO):

• Ask for "papers", certification, or proof of training

• Require your service dog to wear a vest (although it makes for far less trouble if your dog does wear one)

• Deny access based on a dog's breed or size

• Deny access to food establishments

• Ask if your dog is a service dog required because of a disability when it is obvious that it is (you are in a wheelchair or are blind and use a guide dog)

• Ask about the nature of your disability

DEALING WITH PEOPLE

If you have handled a service dog before you already know how much attention it can bring when you are in public. (Especially if your service dog is exceptionally fluffy or tiny).

Another surefire way your service dog will attract attention is if it is an unusual or controversial breed.

If this is your first time handling a service dog, prepare yourself for all of it. Do the role-playing exercise in this workbook to practice how to answer ridiculous questions.

People, adults even, will also come up and try to pet your dog. It does not seem to matter much to them if the dog's uniform clearly states "Do not touch".

Maybe in other parts of the US people, in general, are more educated on proper service dog etiquette, where I live is primitive in that sense and people are mostly clueless.

People will also try and get your dog's attention using kissy noises, a high-pitched voice, or sometimes even food.

Kids often run up delighted to see a dog and invade you and the dog's boundaries. Sometimes parents even get offended when you ask their child not to pet your service dog.

You will be bombarded with questions and statements like "I didn't know you can bring dogs in here."

One I hear frequently is, "Does he bite?" Well of course he doesn't bite, I am thinking. What they actually mean is that they want to pet the dog and have no idea that they should not distract a service dog.

If your disability is "invisible", having a service dog will bring attention to the fact that you do have a disability. You will also get people asking you questions about the dog you are training, assuming you are training it for someone else.

Plan in advance for all of these questions and think of how you might deal with them.
I do come across some people who do ask if they can touch my dog. I always smile and thank them for asking, but that my dog is working (or in training).

I get anxious with access challenges and people constantly asking me questions but that doesn't mean that is the case for everyone.

I had a client who had cerebral palsy and was in a wheelchair. He was a really smart and sociable guy but being in a chair with a disability, people tended to ignore that he was even there.

When we trained his service dog, Buddy, it was an entirely different thing. Buddy became an ice breaker and people now would approach the team and spark up a conversation. For my client, this was great.

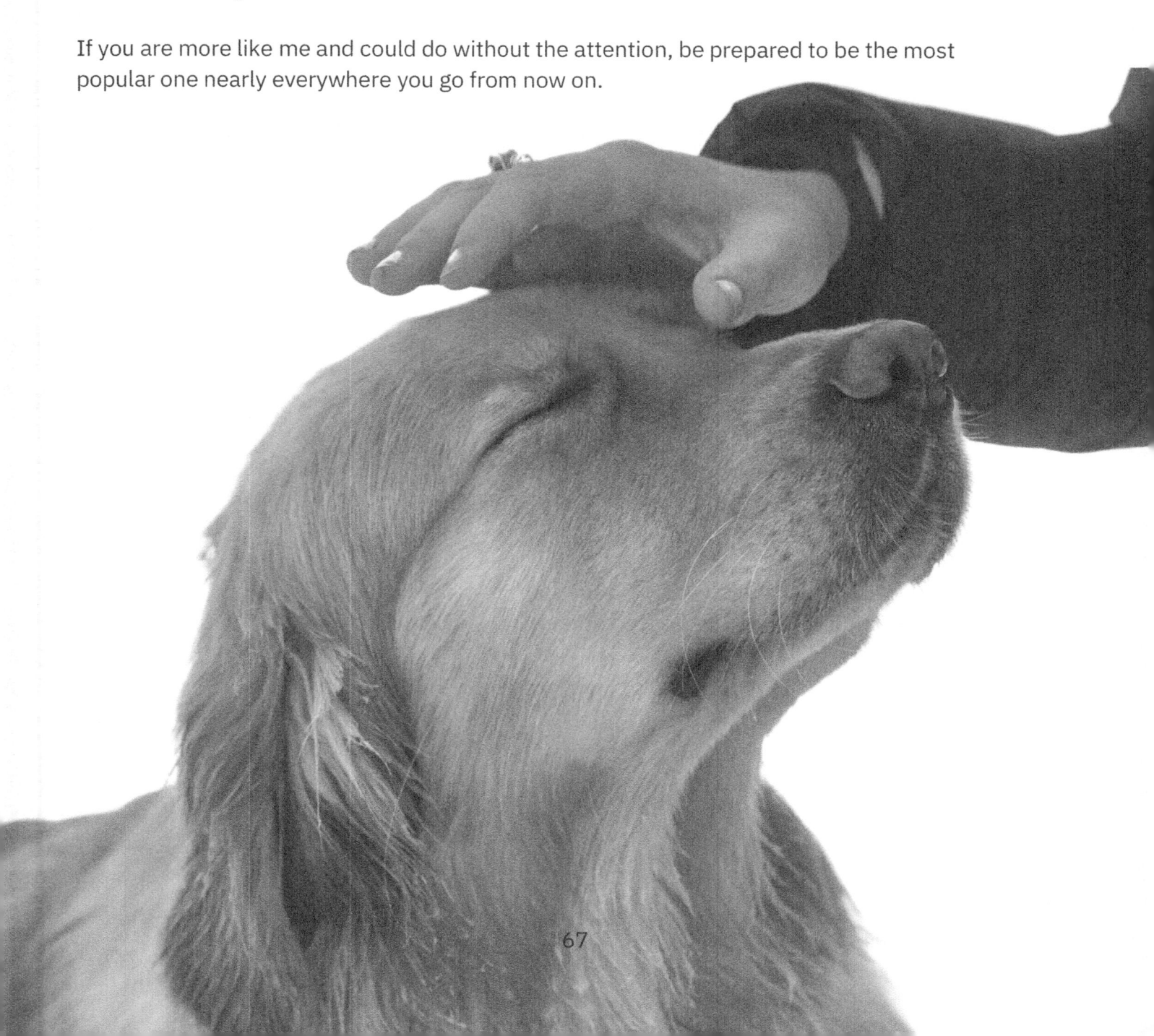

If you are more like me and could do without the attention, be prepared to be the most popular one nearly everywhere you go from now on.

YOUR ROLE AS THE EDUCATOR

By handling a service dog, you take on the role as an educator by default. There are very few laymen who know the rules under ADA (or DOT, HUD etc.)

Business owners SHOULD know and should educate their employees on the basics, but this rarely seems to happen.

People are often in disbelief at how the ADA law states our rights as people with disabilities who choose to handle a service dog.

Many times, they assume they know. They insist that service dogs must have papers that handlers carry with them and will not listen to reason if you try and tell them differently.

It is not recommended in the service dog community to present an ID badge. These can be purchased online; however, there are a couple of issues that arise from these.

First, the companies that sell these are also sometimes selling "certifications" for service dogs. These are scams and anyone can buy them. These scams make a good deal of money by selling fake and unnecessary documentation.

This brings me to the other issue. Since anyone can buy them, people who want their pet to come with them buy them and when asked for papers, they present this to the employee who is challenging them. This further reinforces the idea that we are required to present proof.

Instead, it is better, and I think essential, to carry a stack of ADA law cards that state a simple and short explanation of what they are allowed to ask and where they can contact if they have questions.

I designed several specialty cards for several breeds and some that have just a little bit of attitude. The purchaser prints them out themselves at home. These are for sale for a few dollars on etsy.

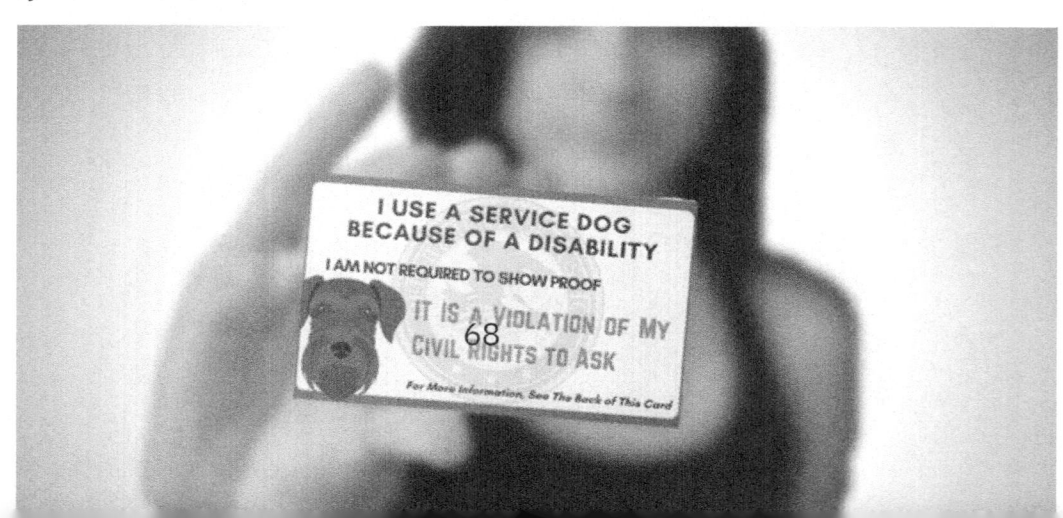

FAKE AND UNTRAINED SERVICE DOGS

CAN YOU SPOT THE DOG THAT IS NOT A SERVICE DOG OR AT LEAST HAS NOT BEEN TRAINED TO A PUBLIC ACCESS LEVEL OF TRAINING RIGHT AWAY?

It is usually the one looking super stressed and:

- Paying much more attention to people other than the handler
- Straining at the leash
- Barking and lunging at another service dog
- Often, but not always, it is a small dog
- Might be riding in the cart
- Sniffs displays at will
- May lift a leg in the store without the handler noticing
- Whose handler answers the question "What task does your dog do?" by saying the dog "calms them down"
- Does not seem to follow any directions the handler gives it

Don't be this guy. It is becoming a problem for businesses and service dog handlers more and more often for several reasons.

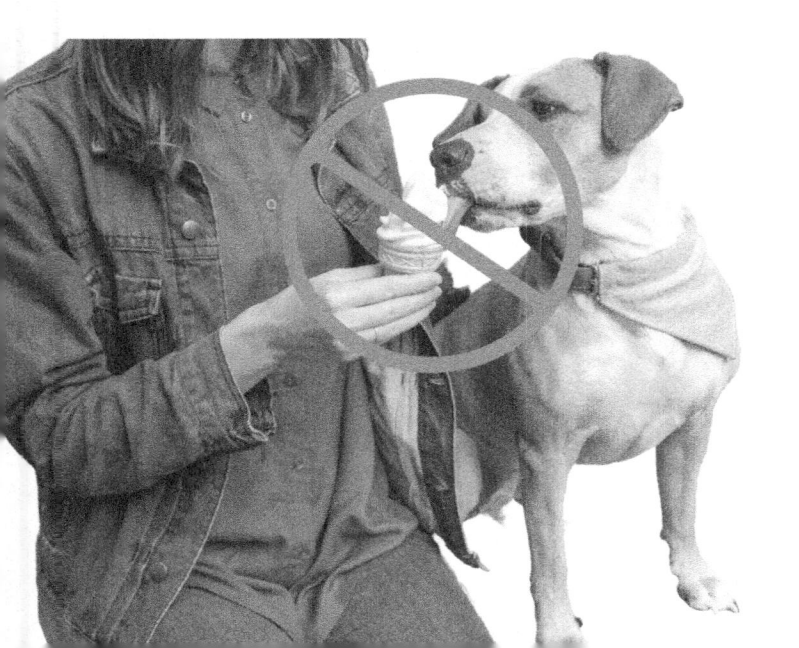

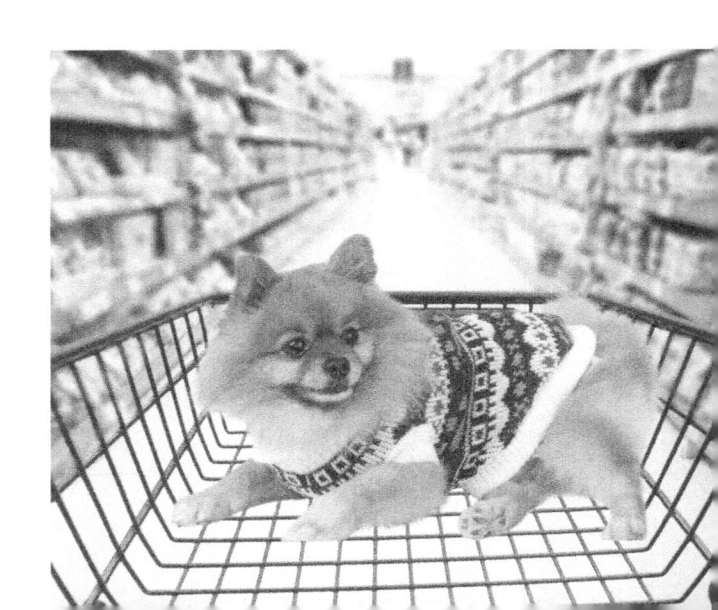

OF COURSE, THERE ARE OBVIOUS REASONS:

• It is now against the law to misrepresent a dog as a service dog

• It is unethical for someone to lie about being disabled to bring their pet into a business or fly them for free

• An increasing number of online companies are making a profit by selling vests and unnecessary registration "papers" to people who want their dog "certified" as a service dog so they can take their pet with them and avoid pet fees

• It pisses people off who have actually put in the hard work training their service dog because they legitimately need it to help them with a disability

However, it is even more so becoming a problem for people with disabilities who either have a service dog or may want to handle one in the future

THESE ARE SOME OF THE REASONS WHY:

• Businesses and their employees are completely confused about what the law actually states. Most employees are never trained in what they are allowed to ask a service dog handler and if they are aware of the right questions, they have no idea what the correct answer should be

• Legitimate service dog handlers know that we should never provide "papers" or an ID badge when a manager or employee demands it because that would further reinforce the mistaken belief that we are required to provide it. Handlers who are not disabled or whose dog is not a service dog often purchase these from an online scam company and flash them at will, making it much more difficult for the authentic handler the next time they enter the establishment and do not produce one

• It is extremely distracting and sometimes downright dangerous for a trained service dog to encounter an un or under-trained dog in a store. The dog may distract it from paying attention to medical cues it needs to focus on for the handler's safety and it happens too often that the dog actually tries to attack a legitimate service dog! Trained service dogs and disabled handlers have been injured or traumatized in similar situations.

• We will eventually lose rights as lawmakers try to figure out how to fix the issue. Ideas for solutions include requiring that service dogs only be trained professionally and certified, with a more universal form of proof, and more intrusive screening protocols

• Badly-behaved dogs being represented as service dogs create bias and judgments when they are in public and do things our service dogs have been trained extensively NOT to do

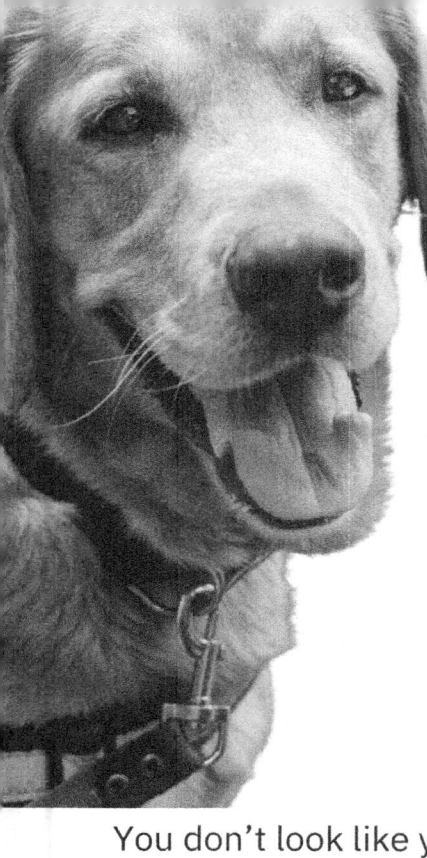

BE PREPARED; LET'S ROLE PLAY CHALLENGES WITH PEOPLE

What would you say in the following situations? It is a good idea to practice how to talk to the public so that when you are asked awkward questions, you are prepared with an appropriate response.

Always remember that not only are you representing yourself, you are also representing service dogs in general. How you interact with a person will partially determine how they react to those with service dogs in the future.

You don't look like you need a service dog

How did you get that vest? I need to know where to buy one so I can bring my dog into the stores

"That doesn't look like a service dog "

"Sorry, the store owner is allergic to dogs so you will have to tie him outside"

"No dogs allowed in the restaurant. The health department says so"

An adult starts petting your dog without asking.

CHAPTER 11: TAKING ACTION

FILING A TITLE II COMPLAINT

Title II complaints are complaints against state and Federal governments.

The following information is from the Title II Technical Assistance Manual developed by the U.S. Department of Justice. The manual provides guidance on the regulations under Title II of the ADA.

II-9.2000 COMPLAINTS

A person or a specific class of individuals or their representative may file a complaint alleging discrimination on the basis of disability.

WHAT MUST BE INCLUDED IN A COMPLAINT?
- A complaint must be in writing
- It should contain the name and address of the individual or the representative filing the complaint
- The complaint should describe the public entity's alleged discriminatory action in sufficient detail to inform the Federal agency of the nature and date of the alleged violation
- The complaint must be signed by the complainant or by someone authorized to do so on his or her behalf
- Complaints filed on behalf of classes or third parties shall describe or identify (by name, if possible) the alleged victims of discrimination

IS THERE A TIME PERIOD IN WHICH A COMPLAINT MUST BE FILED?
Yes. A complaint must be filed within 180 days of the date of the alleged act(s) of discrimination unless the time for filing is extended by the Federal agency for good cause. As long as the complaint is filed with any Federal agency, the 180-day requirement will be considered satisfied.

WHERE SHOULD A COMPLAINT BE FILED?
A complaint may be filed with either:

- Any Federal agency that provides funding to the public entity that is the subject of the complaint
- A Federal agency designated in the title II regulation to investigate title II complaints
- The Department of Justice

Complainants may file with a Federal funding agency that has section 504 jurisdiction if known.

If no Federal funding agency is known, then complainants should file with the appropriate designated agency. In any event, complaints may always be filed with the Department of Justice, which will refer the complaint to the appropriate agency. The Department's regulation designates eight Federal agencies to investigate title II complaints primarily in those cases where there is no Federal agency with section 504 jurisdiction.

HOW WILL EMPLOYMENT COMPLAINTS BE HANDLED?
Individuals who believe that they have been discriminated against in employment by a State or local government in violation of title II may file a complaint:

- With a Federal agency that provides financial assistance, if any, to the State or local program in which the alleged discrimination took place
- With the EEOC, if the State or local government is also subject to title I of the ADA (see II-4.0000)
- With the Federal agency designated in the title II regulation to investigate complaints in the type of program in which the alleged discrimination took place

As is the case with complaints related to non-employment issues, employment complaints may be filed with the Department of Justice, which will refer the complaint to the appropriate agency.

WHICH ARE THE DESIGNATED FEDERAL AGENCIES AND WHAT ARE THEIR AREAS OF RESPONSIBILITY?
The eight designated Federal agencies, the functional areas covered by these agencies, and the addresses for filing a complaint are the:

DEPARTMENT OF AGRICULTURE:
All programs, services, and regulatory activities relating to farming and the raising of livestock, including extension services.

DEPARTMENT OF HEALTH AND HUMAN SERVICES:
All programs, services, and regulatory activities relating to the provision of health care and social services, including schools of medicine, dentistry, nursing, and other health-related schools, the operation of health care and social service providers and institutions, including "grass-roots" and community services organizations and programs, and preschool and daycare programs.

DEPARTMENT OF HOUSING AND URBAN DEVELOPMENT:
All programs, services, and regulatory activities relating to State and local public housing, and housing assistance and referral.

DEPARTMENT OF THE INTERIOR:
All programs, services, and regulatory activities relating to lands and natural resources, including parks and recreation, water and waste management, environmental protection, energy, historic and cultural preservation, and museums.

DEPARTMENT OF JUSTICE:
All programs, services, and regulatory activities relating to law enforcement, public safety, and the administration of justice, including courts and correctional institutions; commerce and industry, including general economic development, banking and finance, consumer protection, insurance, and small business; planning, development, and regulation (unless assigned to other designated agencies); State and local government support services (e.g., audit, personnel, comptroller, administrative services); all other government functions not assigned to other designated agencies.

DEPARTMENT OF LABOR:
All programs, services, and regulatory activities relating to labor and the work force.

DEPARTMENT OF TRANSPORTATION:
All programs, services, and regulatory activities relating to transportation, including highways, public transportation, traffic management (non-law enforcement), automobile licensing and inspection, and driver licensing.

FILING A TITLE III COMPLAINT
FROM THE ADA WEBSITE

Title III prohibits discrimination based on disability in public accommodations.

PRIVATE ENTITIES COVERED BY TITLE III INCLUDE:
- Places of lodging
- Establishments serving food and drinks
- Places of exhibition or entertainment
- Places of public gathering
- Sales or rental establishments
- Service establishments
- Stations used for specified public transportation
- Places of public display or collection
- Places of recreation
- Places of education
- Social service center establishments
- Places of exercise or recreation

TITLE III ALSO COVERS COMMERCIAL FACILITIES SUCH AS:
- Warehouses
- Factories
- Office buildings
- Private transportation services
- Licensing and testing practices

If you feel you or another person has been discriminated against by an entity covered by title III, send a letter to the Department of Justice, at the address below, including the following information:

- Your full name
- Address, and
- Telephone number
- Name of the party discriminated against
- The name of the business, organization, or institution that you believe has discriminated
- A description of the act or acts of discrimination
- The date or dates of the discriminatory acts
- The name or names of the individuals who you believe discriminated
- Other information that you believe necessary to support your complaint
- Copies of relevant documents. Do not send original documents.

THERE ARE FOUR OPTIONS FOR FILING AN ADA COMPLAINT:

1. ONLINE

File a complaint by submitting a report on the Department of Justice's Civil Rights Division website.

2. MAIL

Fill out and send the paper ADA Complaint Form or a letter containing the same information, to:

U.S. Department of Justice
Civil Rights Division
950 Pennsylvania Avenue, NW
Washington, DC 20530

3. FAX

Fill out and send the paper ADA Complaint Form or a letter containing the same information, and fax to (202) 307-1197

4. EMAIL

Send your complaint to the following e-mail address: ada.complaint@usdoj.gov

Type of Complaint	Agency to File With	How to File
Employment (e.g., issues at work or in applying for a job)	Equal Employment Opportunity Commission (EEOC)	Follow instructions on the EEOC site
Air travel (involving a specific airline)	Department of Transportation (DOT)	Follow instructions on the DOT site
Housing (e.g., denied housing or denied an accessible living space based on disability)	Department of Housing and Urban Development (HUD)	Follow the instructions on the HUD site

RESOURCES

- **Title II complaint form**: https://www.ada.gov/t2cmpfrm.htm
- **Civil Rights Division online complaint form** https://civilrights.justice.gov/report/
- **PDF Title III form to mail or fax** HTTPS://WWW.ADA.GOV/CRT-REPORTPDF-SEP2021.PDF
- **Equal Employment Opportunity Commission** (EEOC) HTTPS://WWW.EEOC.GOV/FILING-CHARGE-DISCRIMINATION
- **Department of Transportation** (DOT) HTTPS://WWW.TRANSPORTATION.GOV/AIRCONSUMER/COMPLAINTS-ALLEGING-DISCRIMINATORY-TREATMENT-AGAINST-DISABLED-TRAVELERS
- **US Department of Housing and Urban Development** (HUD) HTTPS://WWW.HUD.GOV/PROGRAM_OFFICES/FAIR_HOUSING_EQUAL_OPP/ONLINE-COMPLAINT

Attn: US Department of Justice
950 Pennsylvania Avenue NW
Civil Rights Division
Disability Rights-NYAVE
Washington DC, 20530

(Date)

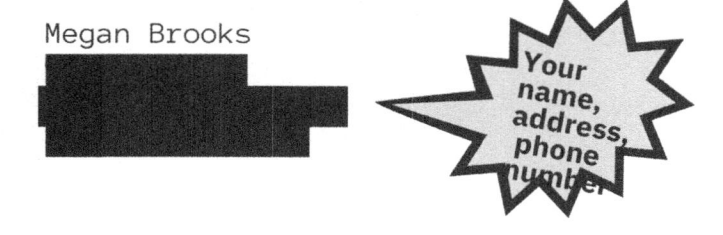

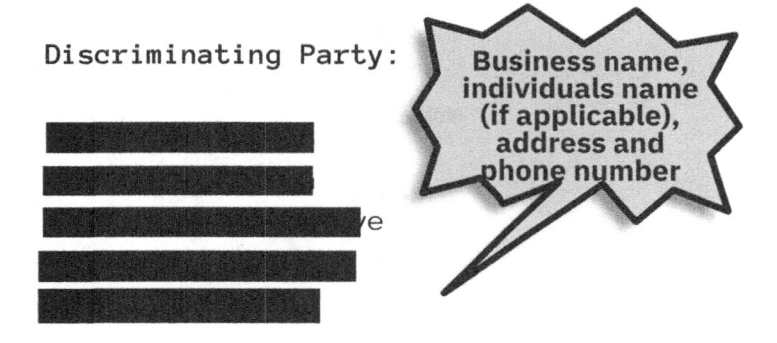

Party Discriminated Against:

Megan Brooks
████████████

Your name, address, phone number

Discriminating Party:

████████████
████████████
████████ve
████████████
████████████

Business name, individuals name (if applicable), address and phone number

Brief but descriptive account of the discrimination that occured

To whom it may concern:

On (date) at (approximate time) I went to (business name and location) with my fully trained service dog.

Upon entering the store, I asked my service dog to down and stay which he did. It was at this time that the owner of the store, ████████████ began to raise his voice at me and told me that my dog is way too big to be in the store and I must remove him. I told him this is my service dog and he then demanded "papers".

I attempted calmly to explain to him the ADA law and even provided him with a service dog card that explained the law.

████████████ took the card but refused to read it. He instead threatened to call the police on me.

Mr. ▮▮▮▮▮ then kicked my service dog out of the store.

Fortunately my friend had accompanied me because I really needed a new phone and we drove 50+ miles to get there.
▮▮▮▮▮ took my service dog out while I finished my business in the store.

I have also attached a letter from my witness, ▮▮▮▮▮▮▮▮▮▮

Wrap up and include any documentation or evidence you collected

Best regards,

Megan Brooks

MEGAN BROOKS

CHAPTER 12:
TRAINING LESSONS

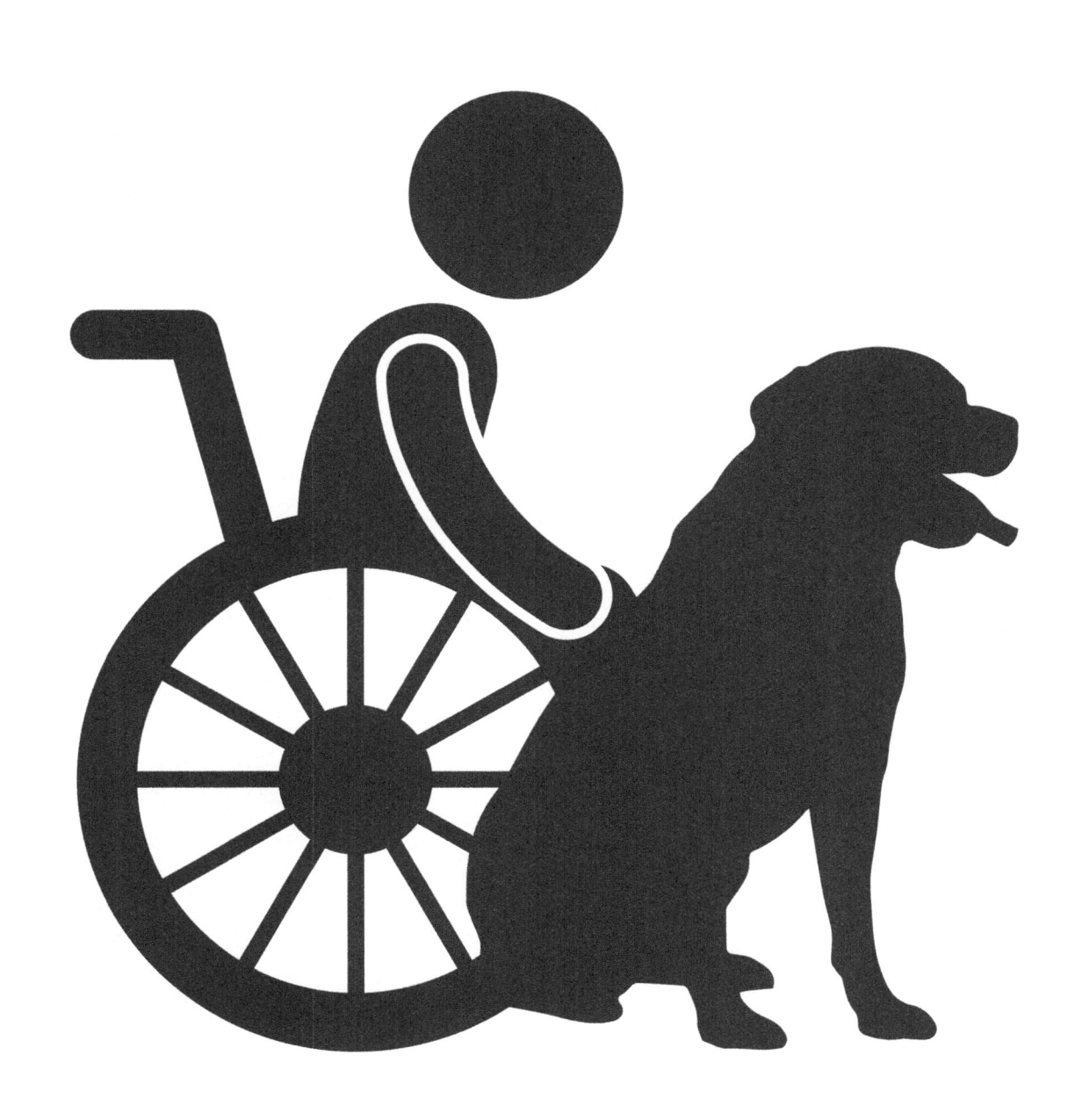

TASK FOUNDATION TRAINING

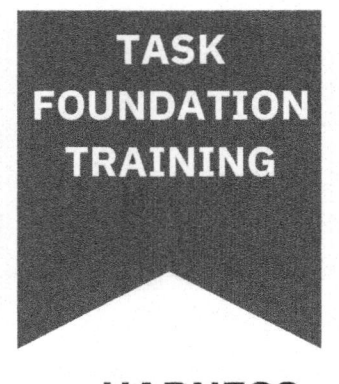

You can begin training with the harness but DO NOT do any physical mobility work until your dog is at least 2 years old

This is the foundation for mobility work such as forward momentum to help you get up or move forward. This can also be used for guide work.

HARNESS TRAINING

1) Train the send out by teaching your dog to put their foot on a target or "mark" on the ground. In this case we will use a frisbee. Your dog only needs to have one foot on the mark

2) Mark, reward and remember to release the dog each time

3) When dog puts a foot on the frisbee every time, you can name it. I use "Mark" or "Point". The dog must stay on the mark until released

4) Start adding distance by walking your dog to the "Mark". Pretty soon, you will be able to start sending them to the mark. Add distance gradually

5) Introduce harness

6) Once your dog is accustomed to simply wearing the harness, begin to put light pressure on the handle. Pull it, tug it and move it around. Reward

7) Walk with your dog while putting light but steady pressure on the harness

8) When your dog is used to walking with pressure against the harness, begin to cue "mark"

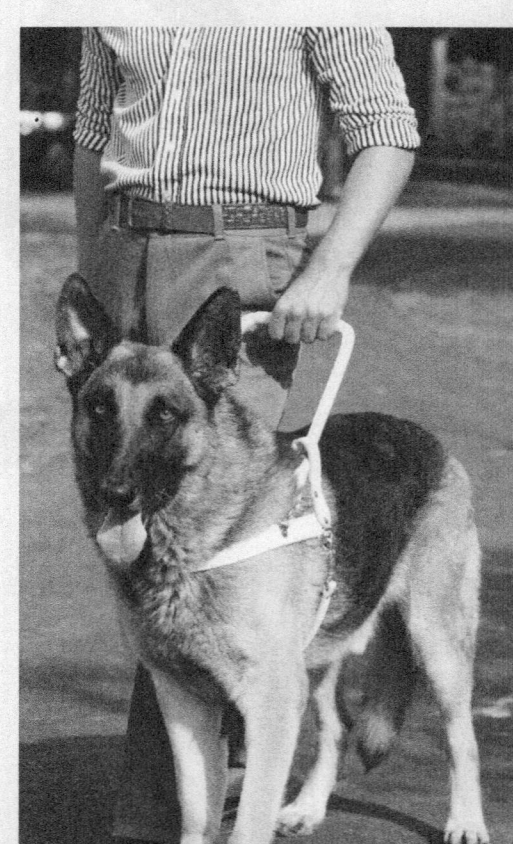

A PERSONAL STORY

Photo courtesy of Bold Lead Designs

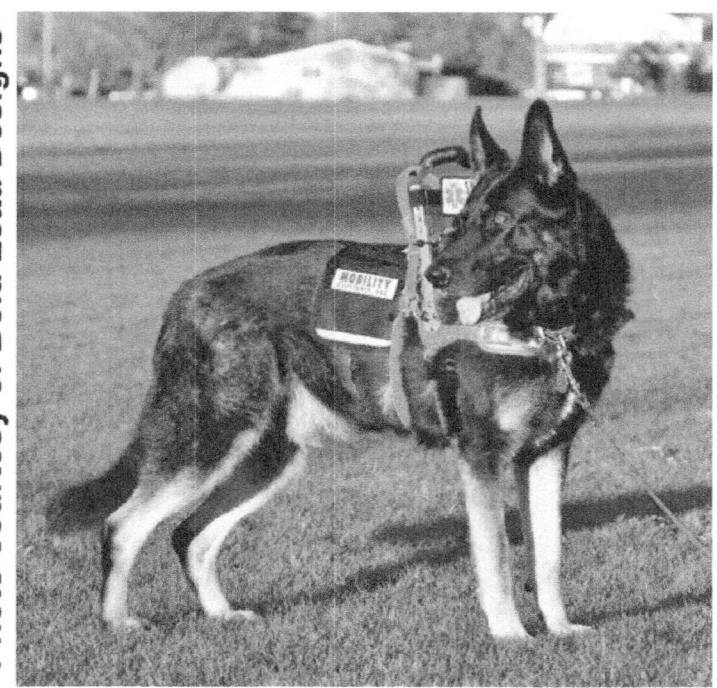

"Kepler"

In 2008, I completed the dog training program and was ready to take on the world. I felt like there were not enough dogs on the planet that were in need of my services to fulfill my passion for training. I lived, dreamed and even spoke dog.

I did not, however, have the first clue about running a business. I needed some help in that area so I signed my business partner/BFF, Mary, and myself up for a class that taught entrepreneurial-spirited women to turn their passions into businesses.

A couple of ladies in class made big, beautiful cakes; another planned events. At least one woman had a housekeeping operation. I was the only dog trainer.

It did not surprise me to be the only dog trainer. What did surprise me was that one of the girls was taking the class because she had created a dog leash and wanted to take this leash to the next level.

The leash was leather and well-made. It had a clip on both ends and a metal ring that kind of free-floated along the length of the leash. She demonstrated to the class multiple ways the leash could be used.

This designer gave me one of her leashes to try out on my service dog, Ramble, who also attended class with me.

It was a nice leash and I used it for quite some time, although I don't think I ever used to it's full potential.

One day I ended up leaving the leash at the park or somewhere and I was bummed because it was a nice leash and now Ramble did not have a leash at all.

I got over it and as time went on I forgot about the leash and the quiet girl from class who made it.

Fast forward 14 years or so and I began to notice service dogs that wore these beautiful leather harnesses. When I would see one, I was pretty sure they all had come from the same place.

Then I started noticing the business name that was behind the elegant pieces of canine equipment I would see this businesses name in places such as the resource section of service dog training books, on very well-known dog trainers' websites, in the credits of YouTube videos.

I recognized the business name immediately. Bold Lead Designs.

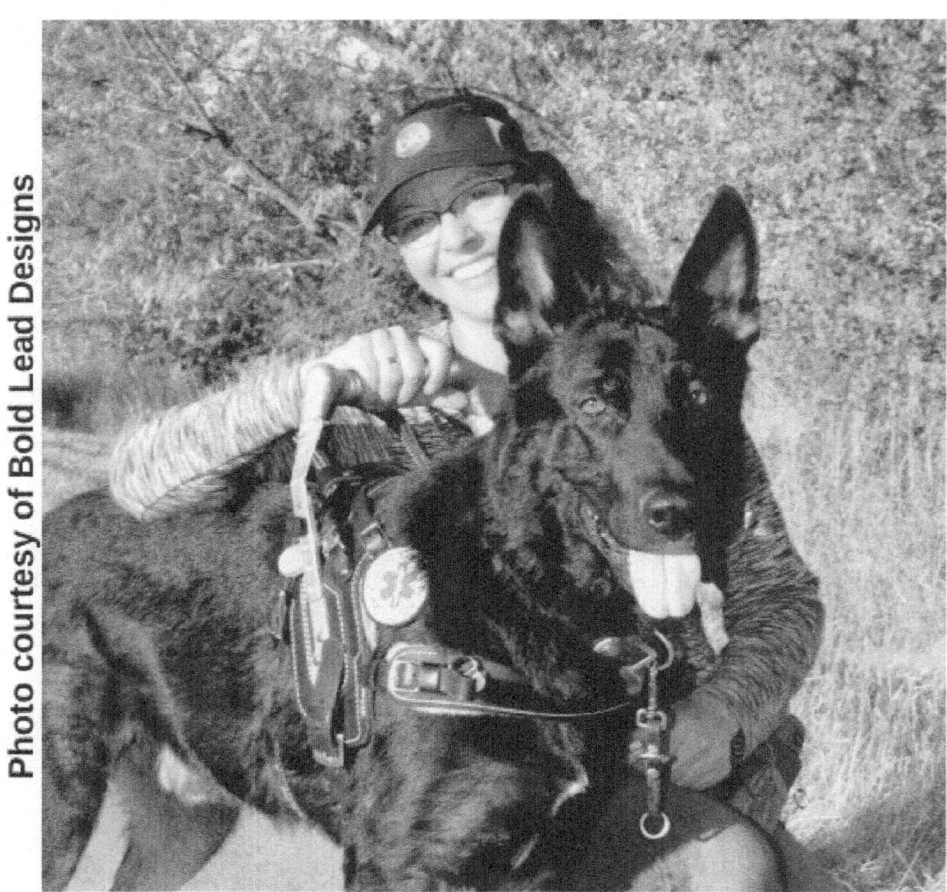

Katrina Boldry and "Kepler"

BLD and founder, Katrina Boldry, are pretty much famous in the service dog world for the custom, handcrafted harnesses and other service dog gear they make. (In fact, they do not only do gear for service dogs, they have a number of other dog products as well).

Katrina had taken what she learned in that class and really ran with it.

The girl with the leash is now the woman behind BLD and they are big. She has several employees working for her and an impressive number of recognitions and awards given to the business. That kind of big.

You may have heard of BLD and you have almost certainly seen their handcrafted work on a service dog somewhere. The designs are absolutely beautiful, they are custom-made to last and pricing is quite reasonable for the quality.

If you have not already checked out Bold Lead Designs, check them out
https://boldleaddesigns.com

Note: I am not an affiliate of BLD nor do I receive compensation for any sale made as a result of my story. I am, however, attesting to the quality and value of BLD if you are planning on purchasing a harness for your service dog.

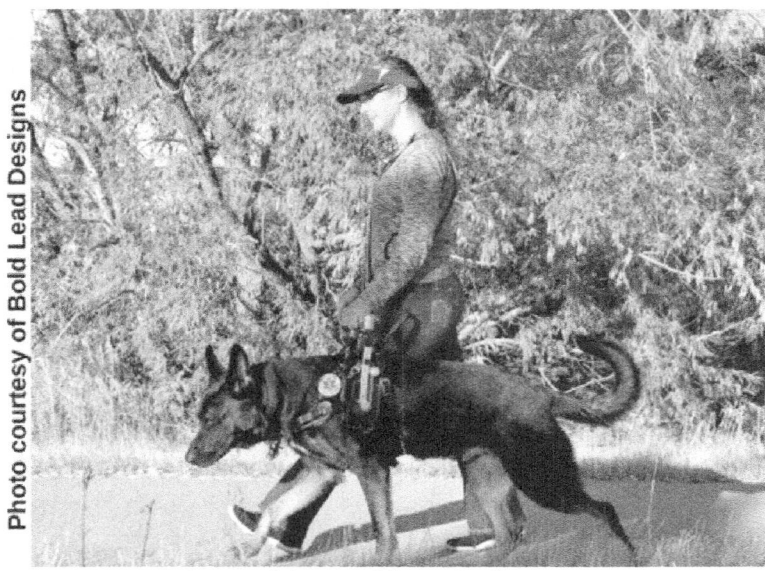

Katrina Boldry and "Kepler"

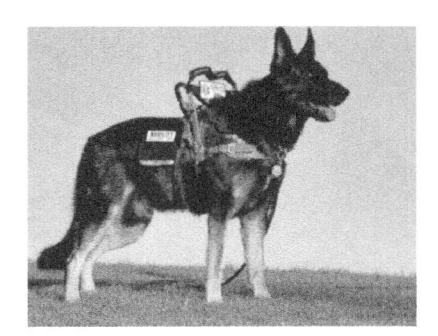

Photo courtesy of Bold Lead Designs

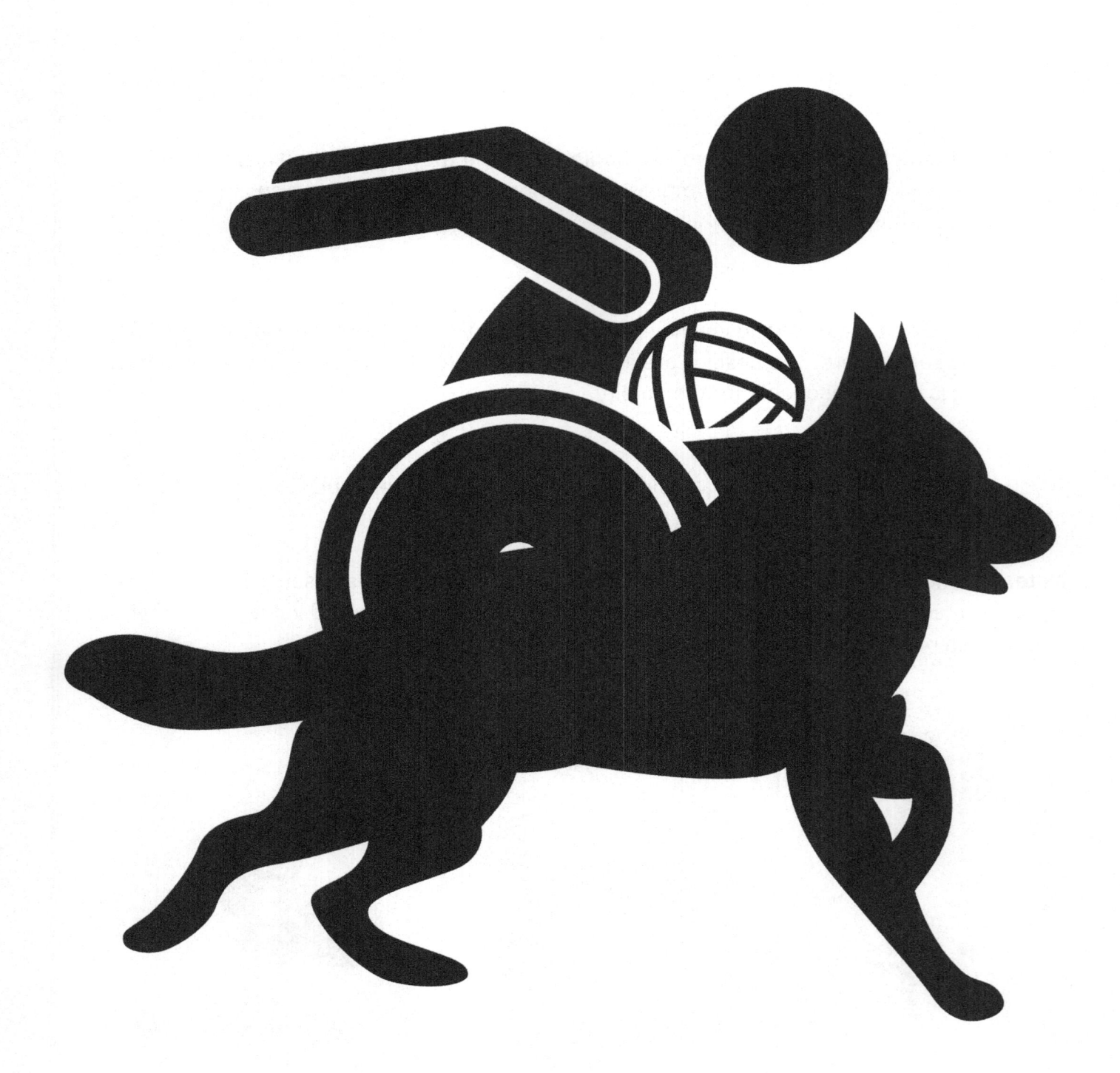

TRAINING ACTIVITY

GET DRESSED

Teach your dog to help make getting ready easier on you by helping to get his/herself dressed

Do not start this skill until your dog can be calm while being leashed for a walk/outing

1.) Hold vest/collar/harness etc. so the part that goes around their chest is in a good size loop

2) In your other hand, hold a treat on the other side of the gear so your dog will have to put his/her head through the loop in order to reach the treat

3) Mark and reward

4) You can remove the harness and repeat, but it may also be more of a reward for your dog to get to go on the outing

5) At the same time, be working on having your dog retrieve his/her gear on cue. When both skills are mastered, chain them together

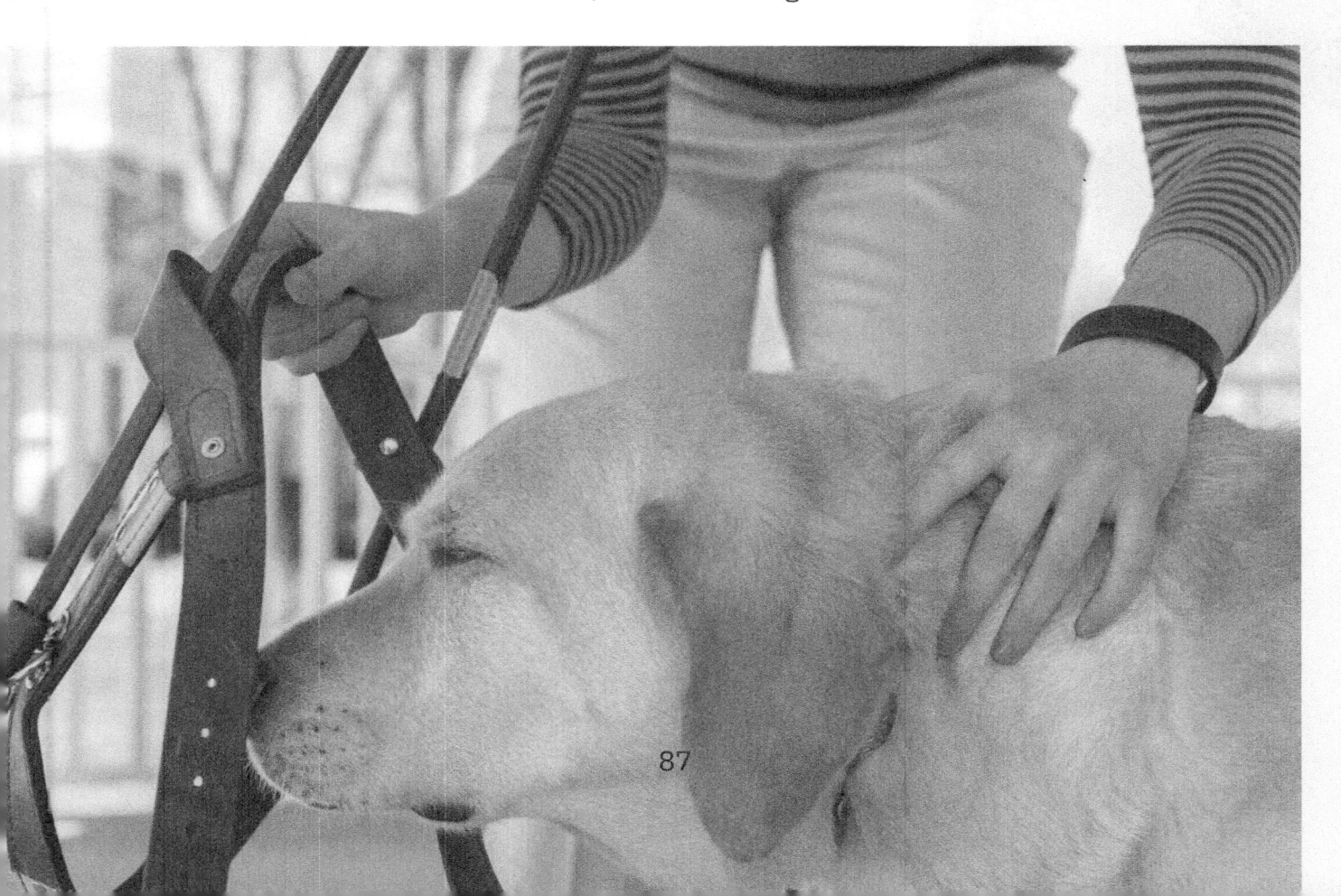

TARGET TRAINING — Target Stick

TASK FOUNDATION TRAINING

Teach targeting using a target stick for either paw or nose. Any stick will work.

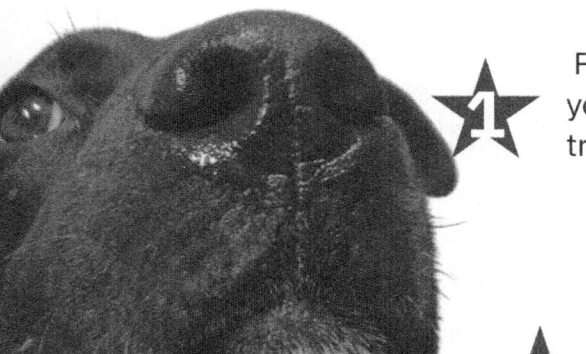

⭐ **1** Put a dab of peanut butter on the end and mark just before your dog licks the peanut butter (the peanut butter is the treat)

⭐ **2** Start moving the target stick around in different places and ask your dog to touch the target on many items and surfaces

⭐ **3** Mark and reward

⭐ **4** Move to Phase II when your dog touches the target every single time, wherever you place it

OTHER ITEMS YOU COULD USE AS A TARGET

- A Yogurt lid
- A strip of duct tape on just about anything
- Sticky note
- Those colorful round dot labels (my favorite)
- A handle from something for a target stick

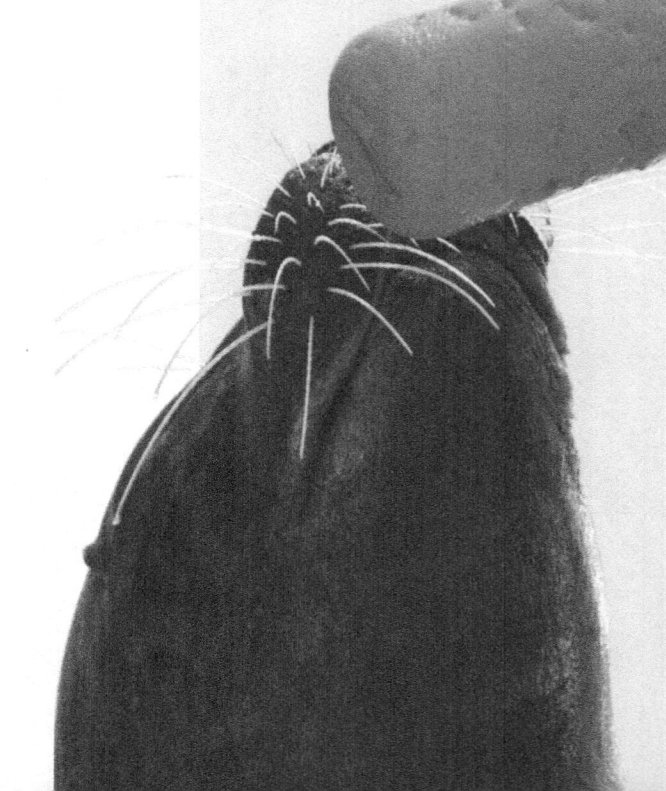

AUTO CHECK-IN/LONG FOCUS

Your service dog must be able to focus on you for an extended length of time. When you go into public, the distractions may be overwhelming if your dog has not first been taught this essential behavior.

THE TRAINING

1. With your dog on leash sit and observe them, but do not talk to or engage with them. You can do this on the couch while the TV is on as long as you can keep one eye on your dog's actions

2. Click or use your termination marker each time your dog makes eye contact. (It should not take long, your dog will be wondering what you are doing) Timing is essential! Make sure you are marking while your dog is looking at you

3. Repeat several times in a row. Your dog can do whatever s/he wants in any position. Pay attention so you can capture the exact moment s/he looks at you, mark and reward the eye contact

4. Do this three or more times daily this week for about 5 minutes

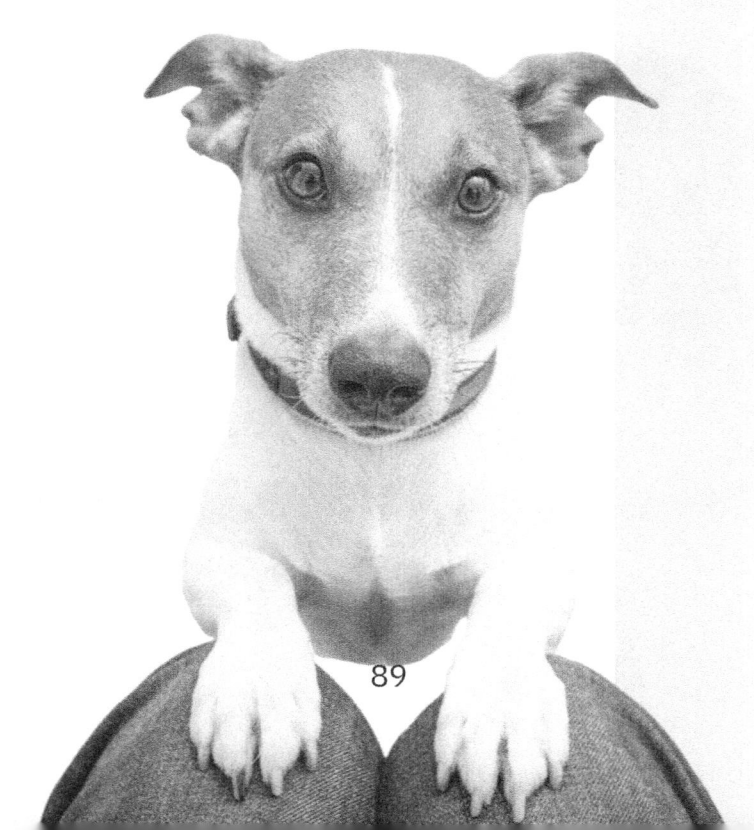

PHASE II

1. When your dog begins to "check-in" on his/her own, try pausing a second or two before marking to see if your dog sustains eye contact for more than one second, when s/he does you will move on to Phase II

2. In the same way as phase I, mark and reward eye contact starting at one second in duration

3. Continue marking and rewarding every second, then extend three seconds

4. Practice often until your dog is able to hold a minute of sustained eye contact with no distractions before moving to phase III

PHASE III
1. Begin at Phase I and begin adding distractions

TIPS
- Use a high-value reward
- From now on, notice when your dog chooses to look at you rather than a distraction and be ready to reward it

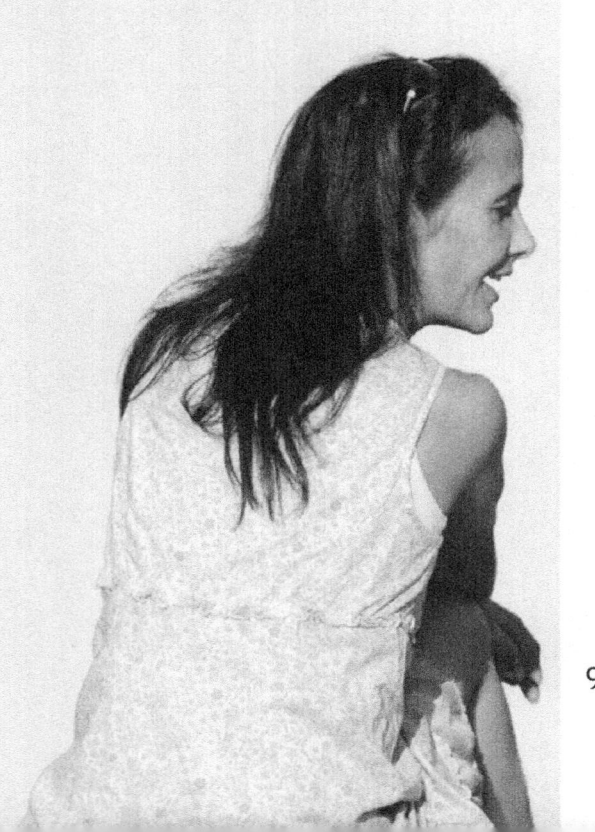

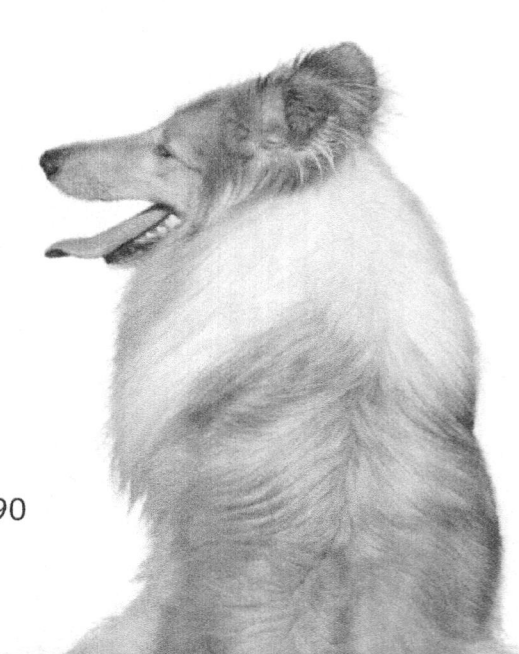

LEAVE-IT PHASE I

1. Place a low-value treat or item on the ground, guarding it with your hand if necessary

2. The second the dog looks away from the treat, you will mark, praise and reward using a very high value food reward that your dog will like (Not the item you told him to leave)

3. Practice using the training sequence.

You are ready for Phase II when you no longer have to guard the treat with your hand.

***Note: Have your dog on-leash when you practice just to avoid them accidentally rewarding themselves with the forbidden treat*

PHASE II

1. Place a low value treat or item on the ground and say "Leave-it"

2. As soon as s/he looks at you, start to back up and use a high-pitched voice, if necessary, to encourage your dog to leave the item and come to you

3. As soon as s/he starts to come, mark (use your termination marker) and reward using a high-value food reward

4. Repeat

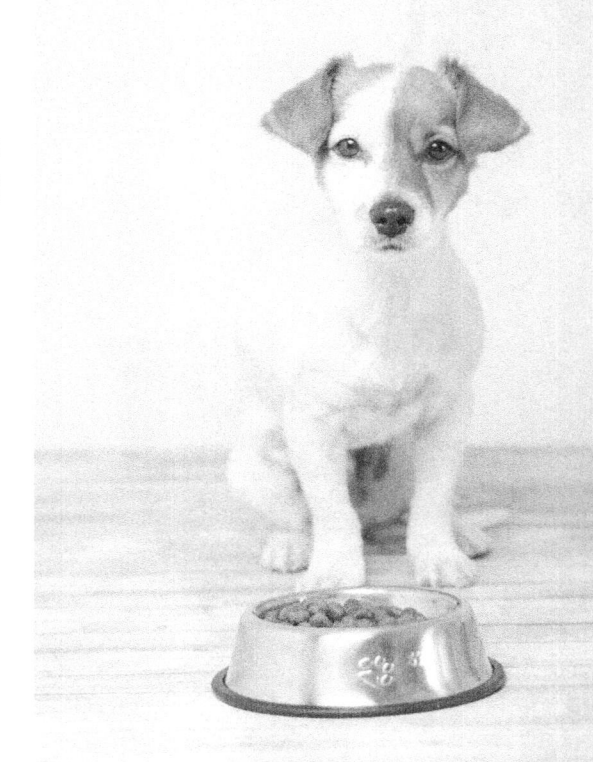

SEND DOG OUT — PHASE I

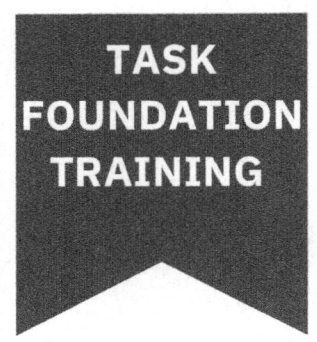

TASK FOUNDATION TRAINING

Being able to send your dog out (distance target) is the foundation for training tasks such as going to find help and for tasks based on sending your dog to bring back an item that is out of sight.

It is the foundation for mobility work essentials such as forward momentum as well as guiding tasks.

I have included two different ways to teach this. One here and the other further on in the book when we talk about harness work.

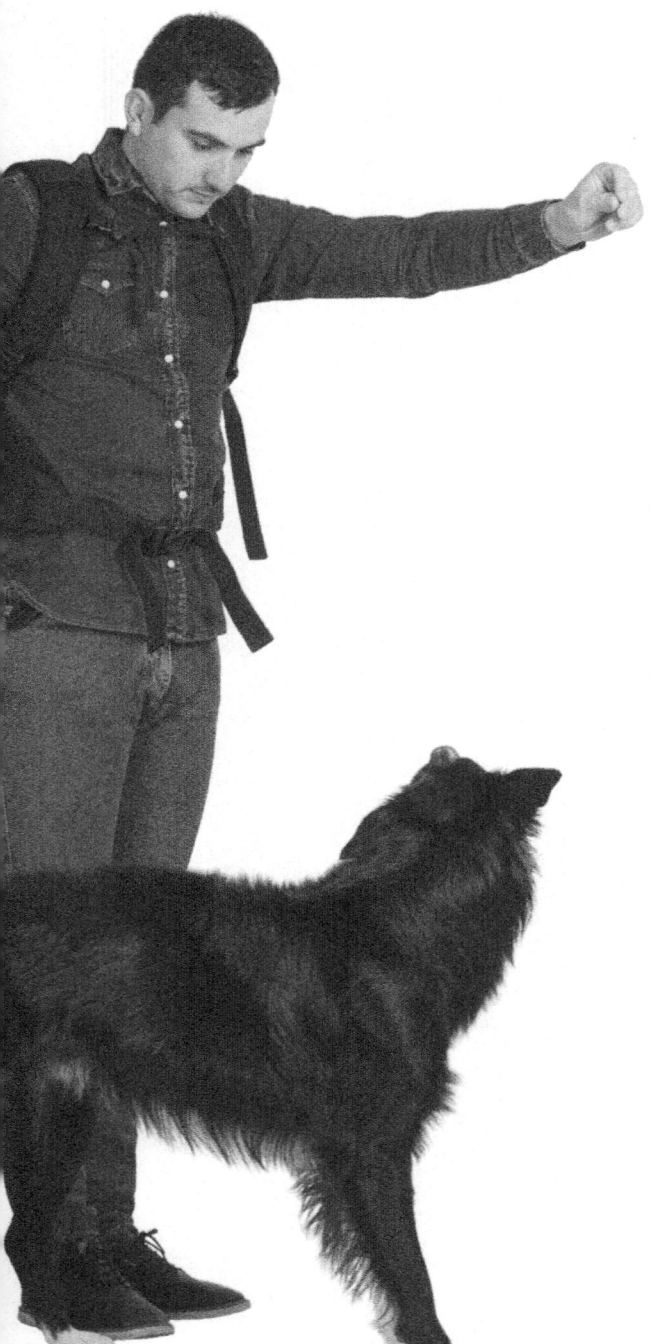

1. Teach your dog to target something larger. An upside down frisbee works well because it is large and more easily seen from a distance

2. Starting about 2 feet away, toss a treat on (in) the target

3. Allow your dog to retrieve the treat, but mark (click) when your dog is on the way to the target

4. Repeat using the lesson training sequence

5. Add distance

PICK UP THE LEASH

Teaching your dog to pick up the end of the leash and give it to you should you drop it could be helpful if you use a wheelchair or if your condition makes gripping things difficult.

Note: This would not be considered a task on its own but could make life easier for you.

DIFFICULTY: EASY TO MODERATE

PREREQUISITES:
Take It   Hold   Give   Bring It   Targeting (stick or laser target)

PHASE I

1. With the leash attached to your dog's collar and while you are sitting down, present the handle of the leash to your dog and practice asking the dog to "Take it" and "Give it"

2. If your dog is willing to do this, practice "Take It" and "Bring It" from the floor by dropping your end of the leash and pointing to the leash handle using a target stick or laser pointer target.

If your dog is reluctant to take the leash from your hand, begin shaping from the very beginning and mark the tiniest of interaction such as a glance. It might help to attach half of a tennis ball or something your dog likes to pick up

3. When your dog is reliable at 90% in retrieving the leash when you drop it, move to phase II and add the verbal cue

4. Begin dropping the leash at random, first with no distractions (in the house) and gradually begin in other places (outside on a walk) with more distractions

5. Mark and reward many repetitions until your dog will eagerly pick up the end of the leash for you every time, even without your cue once they notice it has dropped

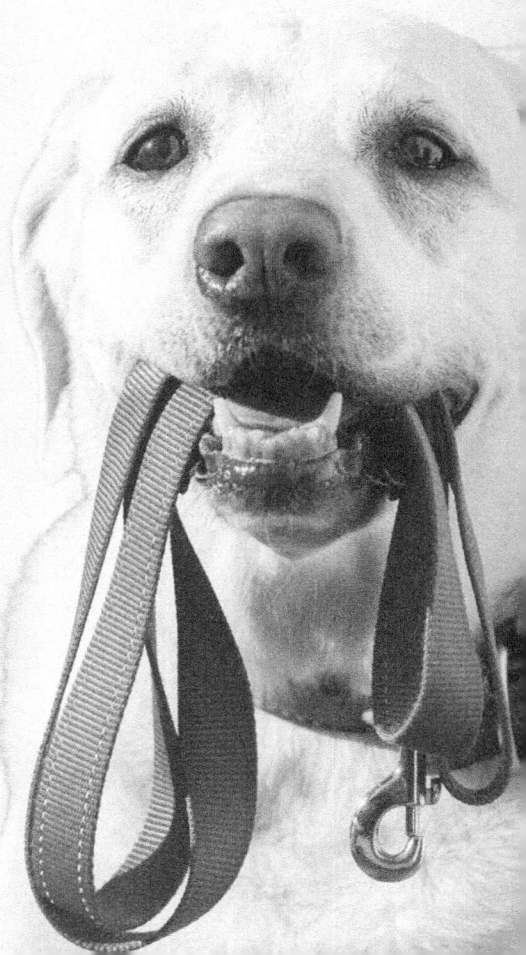

UNDER PHASE I

Teach your dog to lay out of the way at restaurants

★1 Set a table up in the middle of the room (instead of next to a wall) with one chair. Sit in the chair with your dog on one side, on-leash

★2 Lure your dog under the table using a food reward

★3 Mark and reward

★4 Release and repeat using the lesson training sequence

Phase II

★1 When dog is comfortable going under the table, cue "Down"

★2 Mark and reward

★3 Release and repeat using the lesson training sequence

Phase III

★1 Cue "Under"

★2 Cue "Down"

★3 Mark and reward

★4 Release and repeat using the lesson training sequence

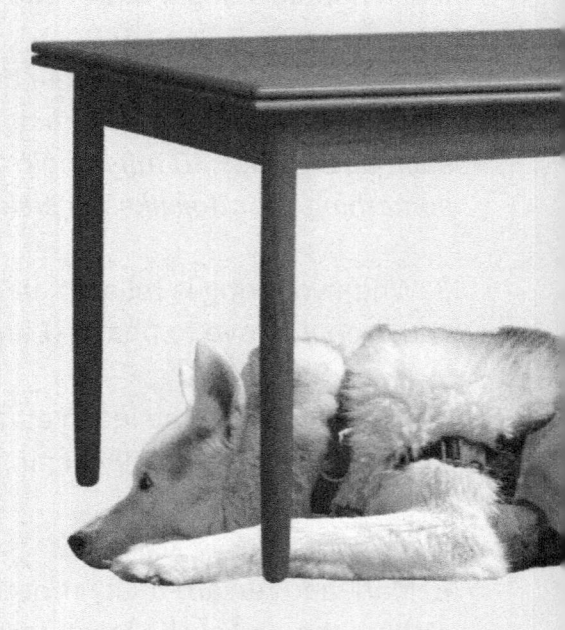

Tips:
Start at five seconds and increase duration.
Generalize at different tables.

FIND AN EXIT

DIFFICULTY LEVEL: MODERATE

PREREQUISITES:
- Send out (distance targeting)
- Forward leading (can help)
- Harness training

PHASE I

1. Start at home, have your dog on a leash

2. Have your dog stay within the house boundary while you let them watch you go a few feet outside of the open door and bait the distance target with a treat. This can be an upside-down Frisbee or even a plastic plate

3. From inside the house, with the target in sight, cue your dog to "send out"

4. Allow them to reach the target and have the treat

5. Repeat using the lesson training sequence

PHASE II

PART A

1. Once your dog is reliable at 90% add the verbal cue. Use something different than what you say that means to go out for a walk or to potty

2. Practice a few times using the verbal cue

3. Now, introduce the harness (avoid having your dog lead using the collar and leash on his/her neck)

4. Since you introduced the new factor (harness) you will step back to the beginning and teach as if it is brand new (repeat steps 1-5 from Phase I, except now you may use the verbal cue)

5. Practice until your dog is 90% reliable before moving to the next step

PART B

1. Once your dog is reliable at 90%, go back and retrain steps 1-5 from phase I. This time you will have your dog lead you using the harness. Start with minimal pressure and gradually increase the amount of resistance your dog feels against the harness

2. When you are reliable at 90%, use the verbal cue you have chosen for "Exit" practice using the lesson training sequence

3. Begin to add distance a few inches at a time until you are several feet away from the door

4. Try cueing your dog to find the exit from around a corner, when s/he does it, JACKPOT!!

5. Remove the target

PART C

1. Once your dog is reliable at 90% at home, begin doing it in each public place. Choose a time and day that are not busy and stay very near the door at first

2. Go back through phase I steps 1-5 until you achieve 90% success

3. When you are reliable at 90%, add distance from the door very gradually

4. Practice often and anytime you and your service dog go through an exit, say the word that you have chosen to label going through the exit

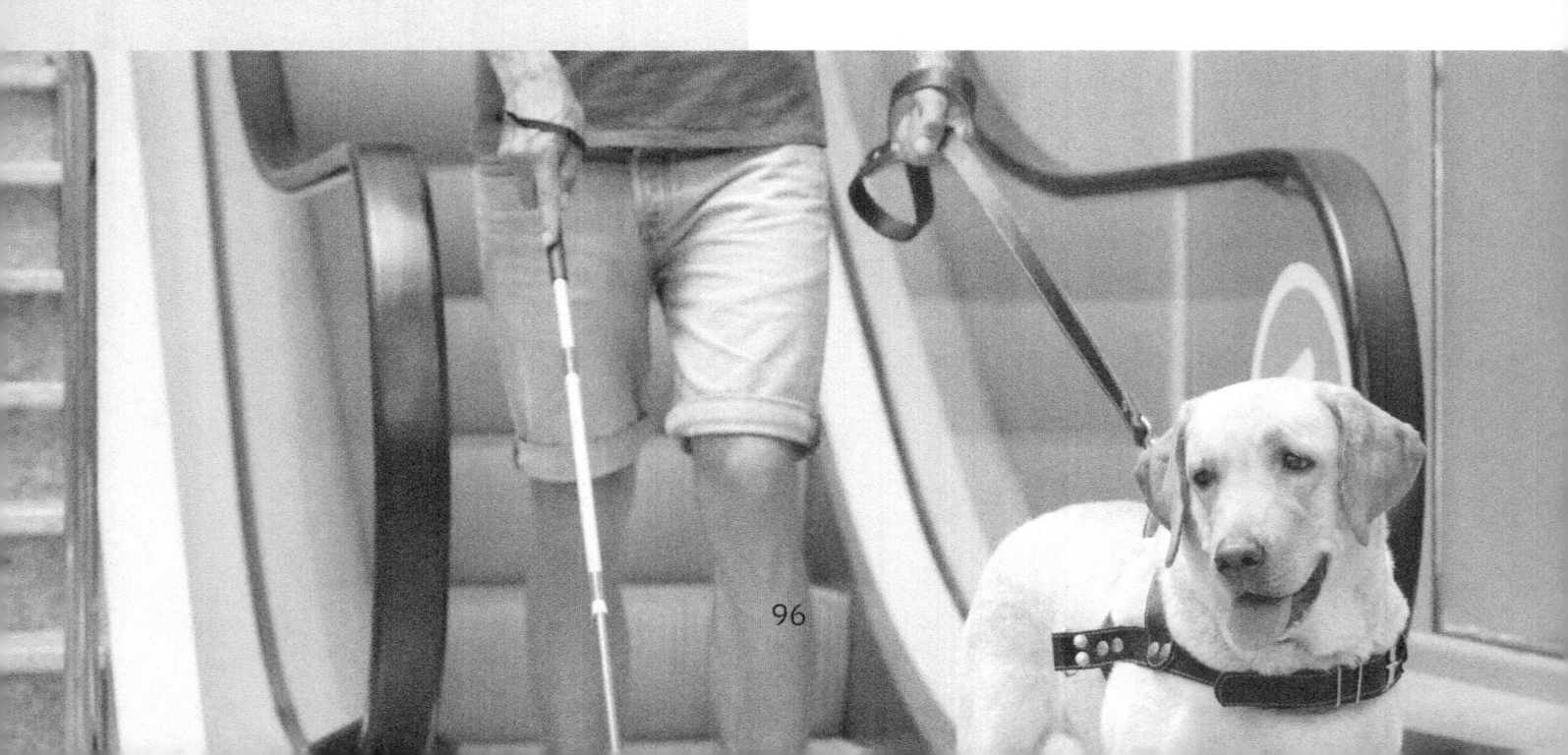

CIRCLE AROUND AND GOT YOUR 6

Crowd Control is helpful for people with anxiety disorders or chronic pain, where bumping people can be painful.

Circle Around is a full circle around you, which creates space around the handler 360 degrees.

Got your 6 is one I commonly train for veterans who suffer from PTSD. This is a stand-stay, most often behind the handler. The dog could also be on either side or in front of the handler. This creates distance/ space between people and the handler.

DIFFICULTY LEVEL: EASY

PREREQUISITES:
- Formal "Heel"
- Pass
- Stand/stay

CIRCLE AROUND

1. With a treat and your dog on-leash in either the "front" or "Heel" position, use the right-hand treat to lure as if you were performing a "pass"

2. Instead of moving back a few feet to give the dog room to turn around beside you as you would when doing a "pass", stay in the same spot

3. Pass the treat to the other hand behind your back, ensuring your dog is following the left-hand treat behind your back and around your left side. If necessary, you can have a treat in each hand and switch hands

4. Go ahead and allow your dog to nibble the treat in your hand a little bit to keep their focus as you switch the treat back into your right hand (with your dog's nose still glued to the lure)

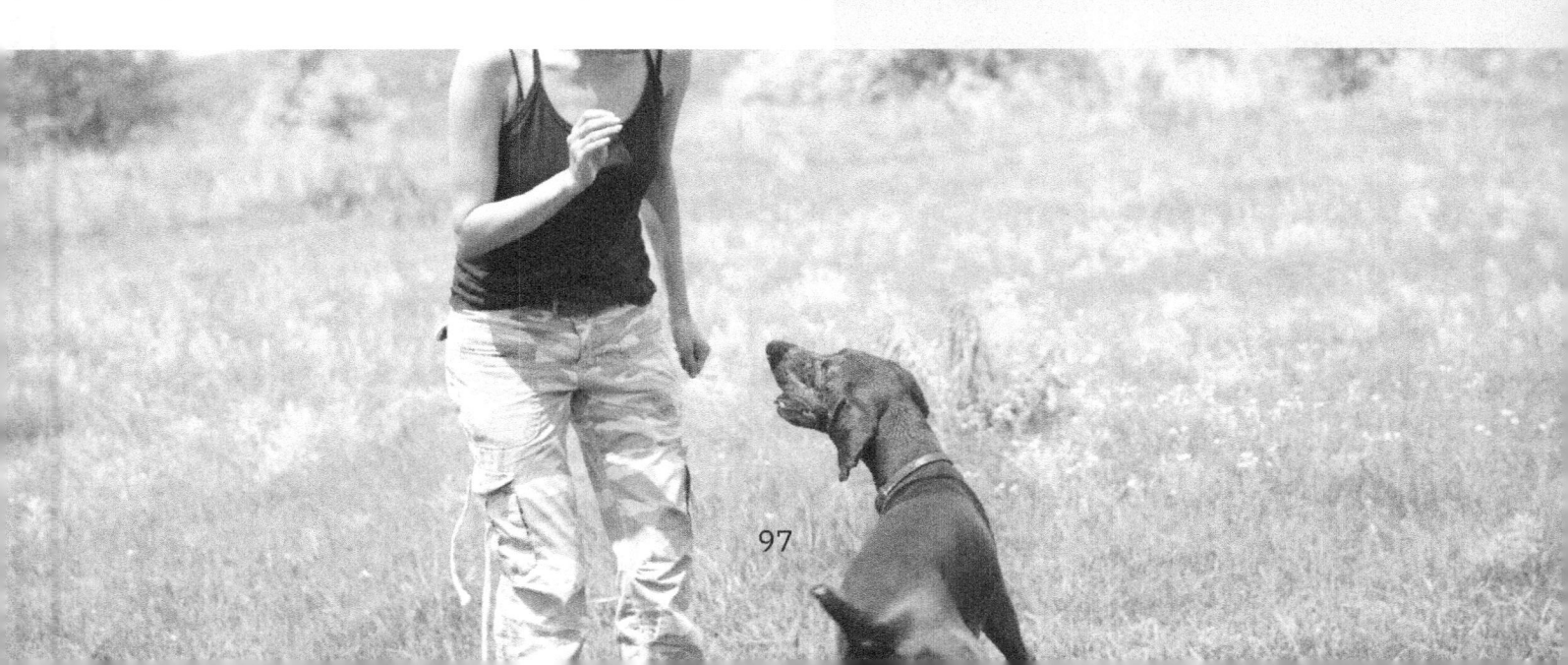

5. This time you may have to move forward a few feet as your dog comes around your left side from behind you if your dog is larger so s/he has enough space to complete the full circle back to the front. Your pointer finger will become your hand signal

6. Release the reward when your dog completes the full circle (it is probably too much to mark using a clicker with both hands full, but you can mark if you use a word or sound you make using your mouth. You can also have a helper click if they have decent timing)

7. Repeat using the lesson training sequence

8. When your dog "gets it" and follows your hand without the lure, begin an intermittent schedule of reinforcement (fade the lure)

9. When your dog is reliable at 90% following the hand signal without the lure, add the verbal cue

10. Train in the opposite direction if you choose

11. Proof by practicing with obstacles (other people or objects) partly in the way of the circle to prepare your dog for crowded or unpredictable environments

- Alternatively, you can use a target stick with peanut butter on it to lure the circle if it is easier for you.
- If your dog is having trouble completing the circle without the lure, mark, and reward halfway through and at the end

GOT YOUR 6

1. Lure your dog into position (front, behind or either side, each taught separately with their own cues)

2. Cue "stay", then immediately mark and reward that position

3. Release and repeat using the lesson training sequence

4. Build duration in 1 second increments

5. Chain the "pass" or "around: /with "Got your 6" together to seamlessly cue your dog to the proper position

6. Add duration and distraction, separately at first, to make sure your dog will STAY in the position

RETRIEVE ITEMS FROM STORE SHELF

You have two options here. Decide if you want your dog to bring the item to you or drop in the basket. In this case, we will have your dog learn to place items directly in the basket. You will teach the dog to drop items in the basket (Part B) first, and then teach the dog to take the item from the shelf next. The final step will be to chain them together.

DIFFICULTY LEVEL: MODERATE

PREREQUISITES:

☐ Targeting   ☐ Formal retrieve (Take-it/Bring/Give)   ☐ Paws up

RETRIEVE ITEM FROM THE SHELF

PHASE I

Part A

1. Choose a low shelf and remove everything from it

2. Place the dumbbell on the shelf. If necessary, you can let it hang slightly off the shelf

3. From a very short distance to the shelf, use a target stick or a laser light target to cue your dog to target the dumbbell

4. Cue "Take-it"

Note: Your dog already has learned to drop the item in a basket that is raised as high as the basket would be at the store. Now that we are introducing new criteria, make sure you go back to the beginning of placing items in the basket by starting out with the basket very close and placed on the floor.

5. Have the basket positioned between you and the shelf. When your dog picks up the dumbbell, cue them to "Bring" the item to your hand, which is positioned directly over the basket

6. Cue "Give-it" and when your dog releases the item, move your hand so it drops in the basket

7. Mark and reward

8. Repeat a number of times

9. When taking the dumbbell off the shelf is reliable at 90%, add your verbal cue. (Placing the item in the basket would have already been trained with a verbal cue)

PLACE ITEM IN BASKET

PHASE I

Part B

Begin adding criteria to the basket part of the sequence first, since it has already been taught with the basket being higher than the floor.

1. Gradually begin to raise the basket an inch or two higher in increments until the dog has his paws up on something to reach it

2. Once the basket is at a realistic height and you have 90% reliability, begin to add distance between the shelf and the basket. When you do this, set your dog up for success by putting the basket back on the floor

3. Once you have mastered your dog carrying the dumbbell 6 feet from the shelf and placing it in the basket on the floor, you can begin to begin gradually raise the height of the basket

4. Once you have 90% reliability at this step, raise the shelf gradually

5. Introduce different items to take off the shelf and place in the basket

Note: It might not make much sense that you would train Part B before teaching Part A, but many behavior chains are easier to chain together when you back chain them.

GIVE CREDIT CARD TO CASHIER

This is a useful task when you are in public. If teaching your dog to give a credit card. cash, or a wallet/small purse to a cahier would help mitigate your own limitations, the steps are outlined below.

This can be chained with both retrieving items from a shelf and placing the items in the basket for a full assisted shopping experience. Way to finally achieve your independence!

DIFFICULTY LEVEL: MODERATE TO DIFFICULT (DEPENDS LARGELY ON DOG'S WILLINGNESS TO RETRIEVE)

PREREQUISITES:
  Solid formal retrieve (Take, hold, bring, give)   Send dog out (Distance target)
                                         Paws up

STEPS INVOLVED:
Take → Send out → paws up   Give (to cashier)   default behavior   paws up
Take (from cashier)   Return/recall → Give →

TAKE ITEM TO CASHIER

PHASE I

Part A

1. Have a partner stand within 2 feet of you and your dog. Have your dog on-leash

2. Give your dog the item (card, cash, wallet)

3. Send your dog out

4. Have your partner give the cue to "give" the card to them. Your partner can trade a treat for the card

5. As soon as the dog receives the reward for releasing the item from your partner, you mark and the dog returns to you to be rewarded

6. Repeat using the training sequence 3 times daily when possible

7. Train to 90% reliability

Do not train the different parts of the chaining sequence at the same time as part A to avoid confusing your dog. Train part A to 90% before moving on to part B. When you begin training part B, you may move on to proofing step A and can change the location you are using which could be helpful in avoiding confusion.

TAKE ITEM FROM CASHIER/RETURN TO YOU

PHASE I

Part B

1. Have a partner stand within 2 feet of you and your dog. Have your dog on-leash

2. Send your dog out, your partner can get the dog's attention if necessary(you are within 2 feet of your partner so your partner can likely just hand the dog the item during this stage)

3. Partner may reward for the recall if deemed helpful

4. Partner gives the item to the dog

5. Recall your dog to you

6. You are within 2 feet of your partner so you can simply cue the dog to give the item to you during this stage

7. Cue the dog to release the item

8. Mark and reward with a high-value treat

9. Repeat using the training sequence 3 times daily when possible

10. Train to 90% reliability

TAKE ITEM TO CASHIER

PHASE II

Part A and B

1. After reaching 90% reliability, (while continuing with no distractions) begin to add distance between your partner and you in small increments

2. Remember to start at the very beginning of training each time you add a new criteria for proofing

3. Add verbal cues if you will be using something other than the formal retrieve verbal cue (take, bring, and give). You may wish to change the verbal cue if you intend to teach the dog to respond to the item's individual name "Toby, go get the wallet"

4. When you achieve 90% at a distance of 5 feet from your partner, add a "counter" low to the ground at first and raise it gradually. (Adding the counter adds a new behavior to the chain so go back to the beginning and work on "paws up" separately if necessary for a while)

TASK TRAINING

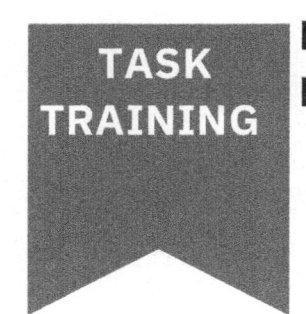

PUSH ELEVATOR BUTTON — PHASE I

This task starts with a paw target. I outline teaching to push an elevator button, but this same process can apply to any push task (light switches, closing doors, drawers the dryer and much more

★1 Teach the paw target using something different than the nose target. I use a target stick for the nose target, so I use a sticky note or a piece of blue painter's tape for a paw target

★2 After teaching your dog to lift his/her paw, place the target on your palm or fist. Present it to your dog down low, closer to their feet. Be ready to mark and reward (use a verbal marker since your hands are full, timing is critical here)

★3 If you haven't taught paw, you can teach from the beginning by marking and rewarding any interaction, such as a glance and shape from there

★4 Mark and reward. Repeat until reliable at 90%

★5 Fade the mark and reward to only reward exceptional (purposeful) attempts. Repeat until purposeful attempts are reliable at 90%

★6 Begin to add height by raising your hand gradually. Gradually meaning 1-2 inches at a time, Go back if your dog struggles

★7 Repeat until the target is at the dog's head height. To teach higher, you can repeat until at the height of your dog's head when standing on hind legs

★8 When you are as tall as your dog can reach on all fours with height, begin placing your hand flat against the wall. Start at the beginning height and move from there

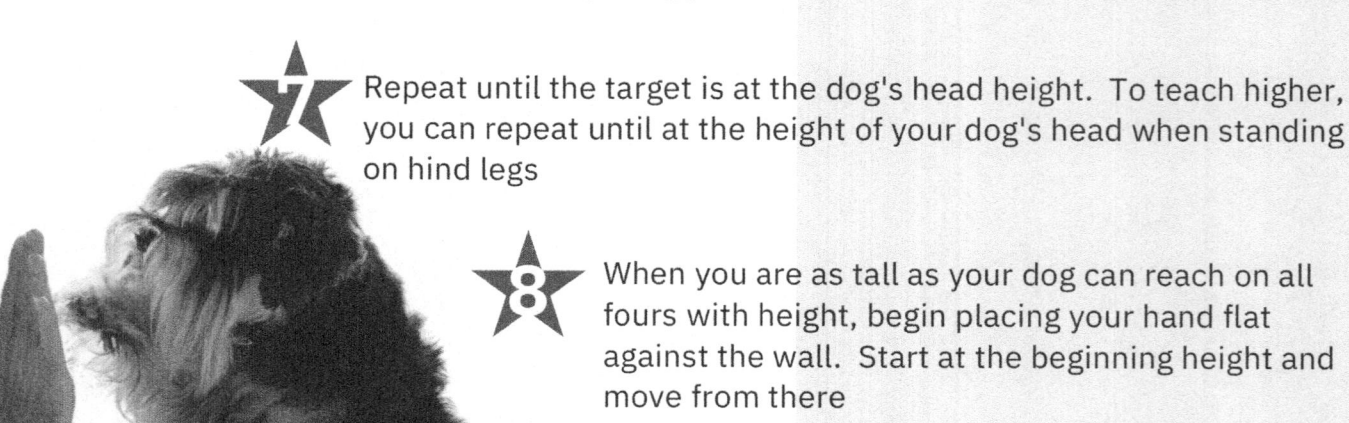

⭐ **9** Repeat until reliable at 90% and then begin to generalize by moving the target to different places and when different locations and heights are solid at 90%, gradually add distractions one at a time

⭐ **10** When step 9 is reliable at 90% add your verbal cue

⭐ **11** Begin placing target on button or item you want pushed. Go back to step one with height and distraction level until 90% reliable at each step

⭐ **12** Generalize to different buttons

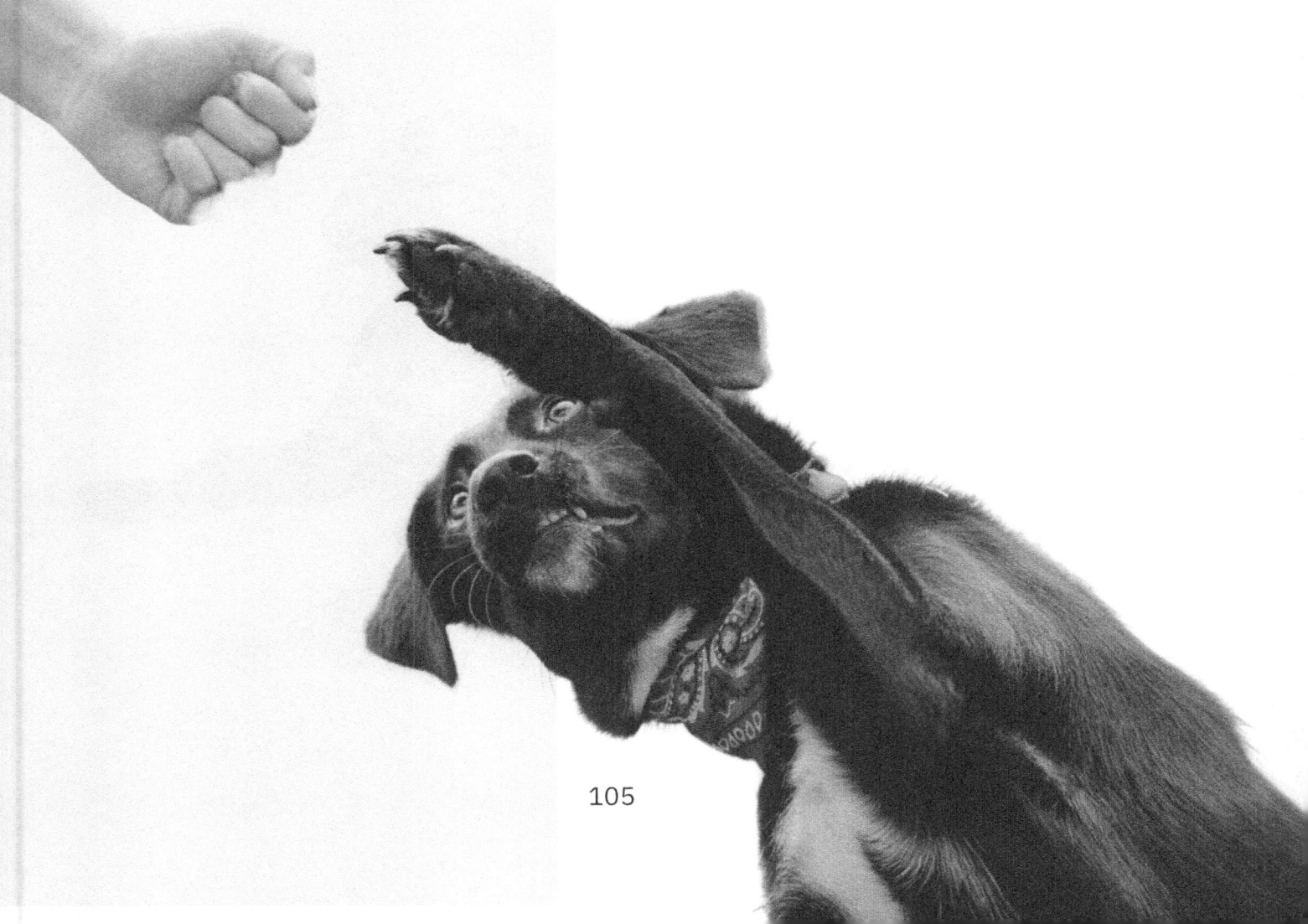

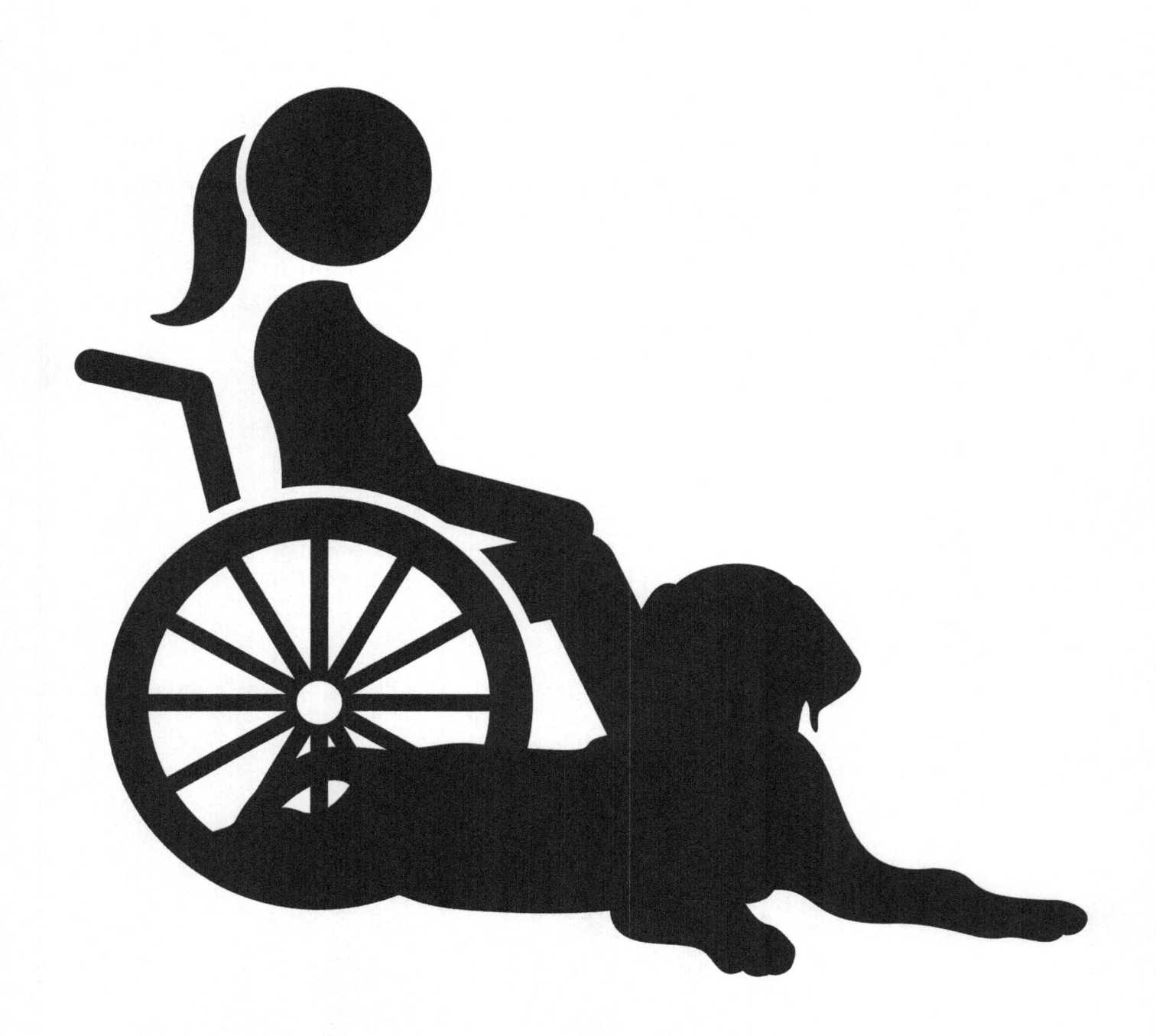

PUBLIC ACCESS FINAL EXAMINATION

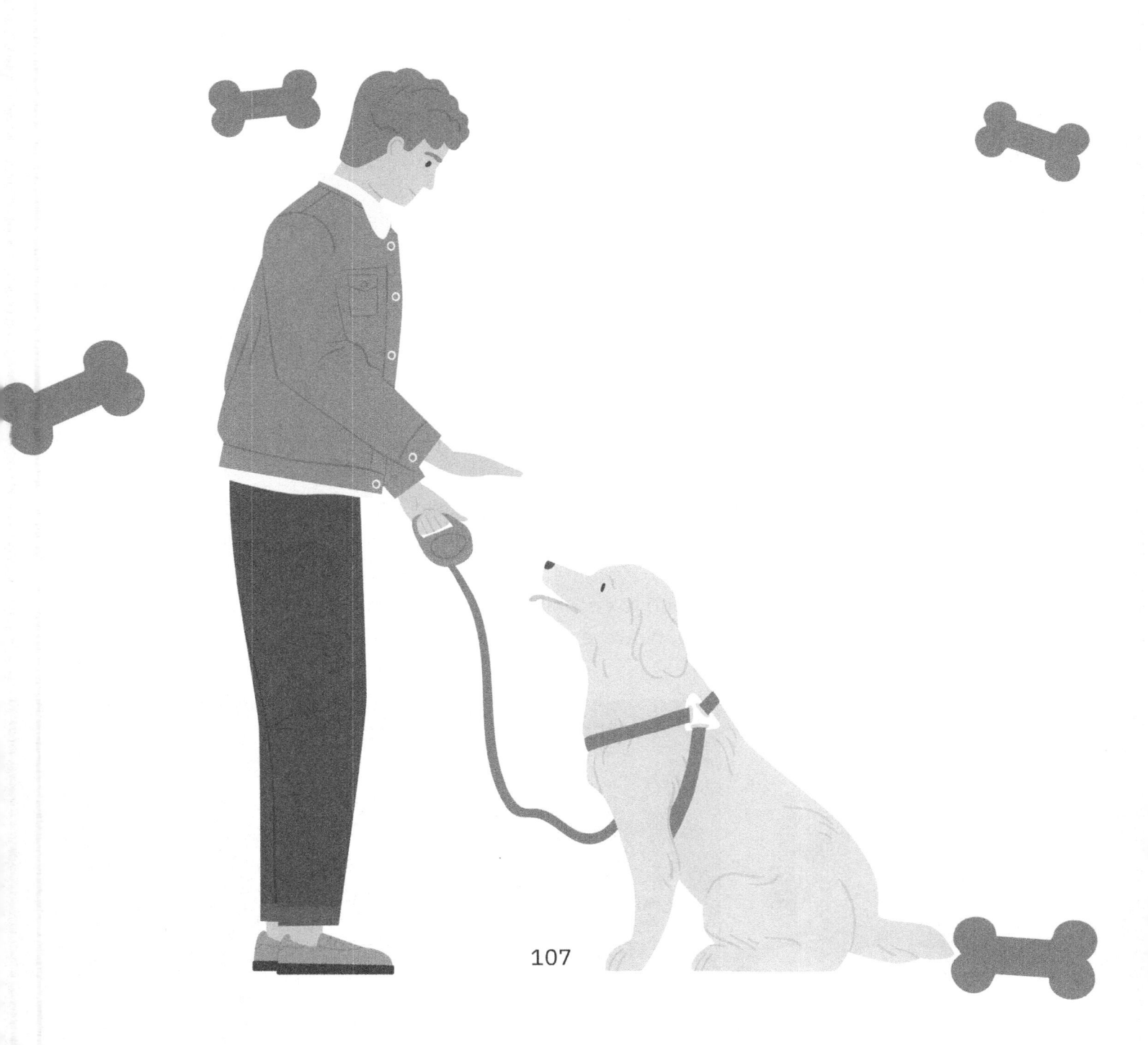

ABOUT THE PUBLIC ACCESS EXAMINATION

This workbook includes a practice test for public access that can be taken as many times as you see fit for your team. The practice test is scored in a way where you can determine where extra training is needed. It can be performed anywhere, public or not.

In fact, the test items will need to be perfected in places out of public first so I recommend using the practice test all during training and in any location.

The *Final Public Access Examination*, while not required by law is recommended in order to hold your team to the highest of standards. It is also a really smart idea to be prepared in the case that you ever do have to demonstrate that your dog has legitimately done the work involved for service dog status.

I hope that it would never become necessary to "prove" your dog is a service dog, but it is much better to be prepared.

In addition, if you file taxes and wish to claim service dog expenses as a deduction, meticulous record-keeping is essential.

I recommend that you video record as many training sessions as possible as well as all of your practice exams and final exam.

Old videos are fun to watch, but it is also very helpful for trainers to watch themselves train.

Issues that can only be noticed when observing from the outside become apparent. If your dog did not respond to a cue, the video may give a birds-eye view of the reason.

You are able to notice things you tend to do while training that you want to change and also things that you do that are working. You are able to see improvement over time.

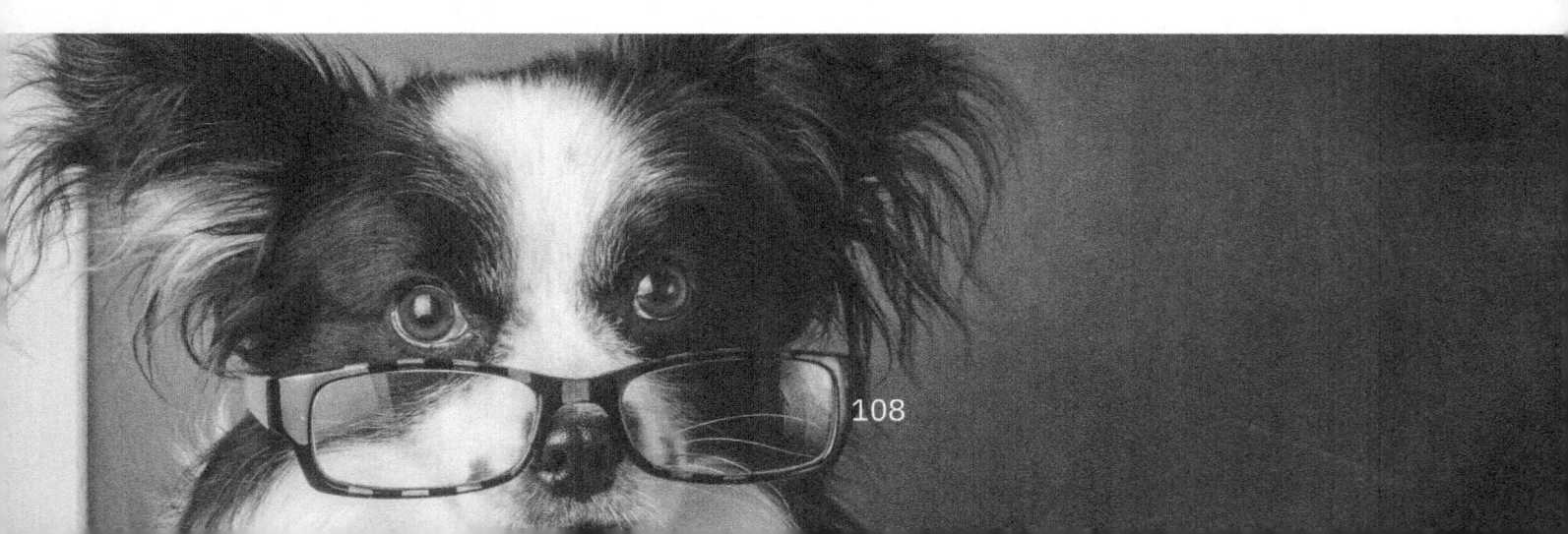

YOUR FINAL EXAM

This public access examination is designed to be evaluated by someone with knowledge of canine body language and has preferably worked with service dog teams (If not, everyone has to start somewhere).

If you have been working with a trainer, ask them to work with you on each portion and to administer the final exam.

You can also ask an AKC Canine Good Citizen Evaluator to perform the evaluation, and there are AKC evaluators everywhere.

Finally, you have the option to do the evaluation virtually and have a service dog professional evaluate your team.

This is a new idea, COVID has made the world so different. (I am programmed to look for whatever growth or benefit can come from any bad situation so this pandemic gave me a lot to work with).

WANT ME TO EVALUATE YOUR TEAM?

If you want me to evaluate your public access exam remotely **for free** contact me!

I would love to be a part of your journey and have your team be a part of my experience.

Contact me if you need help with anything or if you would like to share your service dog team's triumphs, challenges, experiences, and photos (I love photos).

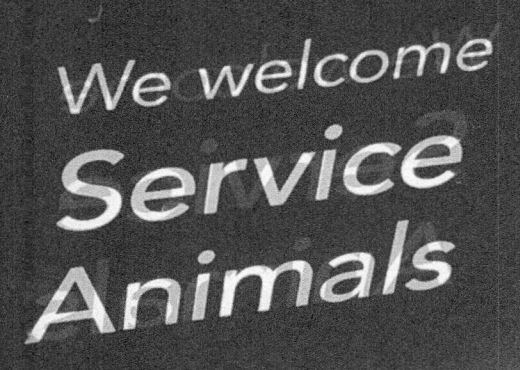

RULES OF THE HPP PUBLIC ACCESS EXAMINATION

The final examination can be administered in any establishment and use public transportation

Training tools that make it possible to work as a team will be allowed as long as the handler demonstrates knowledge of how to use the tool correctly and humanely

Food rewards and electronic collars will not be permitted during the final examination

The final examination will be terminated immediately if the dog shows signs of even moderate stress or if the handler uses harsh correction

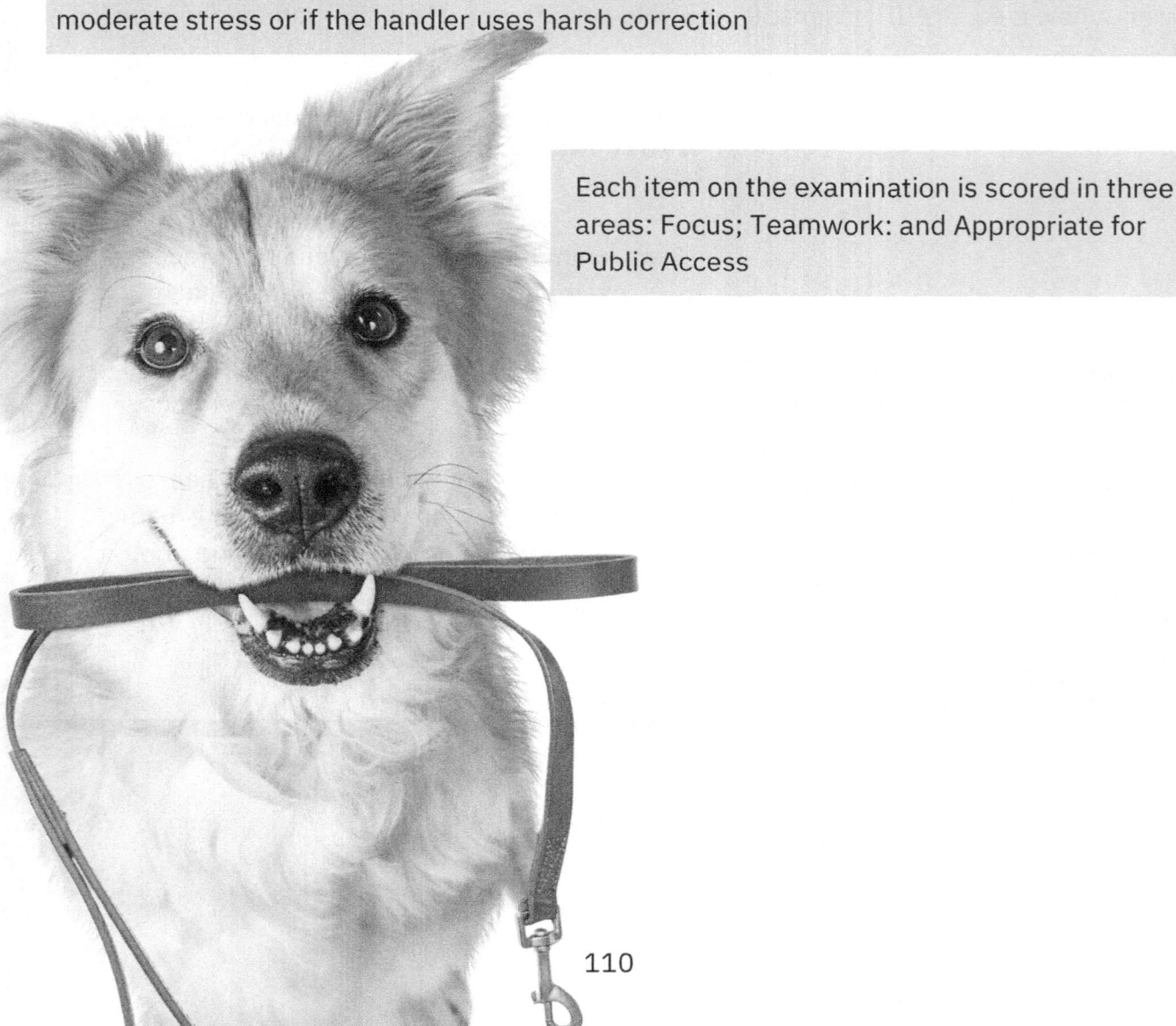

Each item on the examination is scored in three areas: Focus; Teamwork: and Appropriate for Public Access

FINAL PUBLIC ACCESS EXAMINATION

HANDLER:
DOG'S NAME:
LOCATION:

DATE:

---

1) DOG WAITS FOR PERMISSION TO LOAD, ENTERS VEHICLE WHEN CUED BY HANDLER

TEAMWORK
FOCUS
APPROPRIATE FOR PUBLIC ACCESS

SCORE _____ /15   PASS ☐

---

2) DOG APPEARS RELAXED WHILE IN VEHICLE/PUBLIC TRANSPORTATION

TEAMWORK
FOCUS
APPROPRIATE FOR PUBLIC ACCESS

SCORE _____ /15   PASS ☐

---

3) DOG WAITS IN VEHICLE UNTIL RELEASED.

TEAMWORK
FOCUS
APPROPRIATE FOR PUBLIC ACCESS

SCORE _____ /15   PASS ☐

4) DOG SHOWS APPROPRIATE REACTION TO ANOTHER DOG.	TEAMWORK FOCUS APPROPRIATE FOR PUBLIC ACCESS

SCORE _____ /15   PASS ☐

5) DOG REMAINS UNDER HANDLER CONTROL WHEN THE LEASH IS ACCIDENTALLY DROPPED	TEAMWORK FOCUS APPROPRIATE FOR PUBLIC ACCESS

SCORE _____ /15   PASS ☐

6) DOG REMAINS IN CORRECT POSITION AS TEAM ENTERS THE ESTABLISHMENT	TEAMWORK FOCUS APPROPRIATE FOR PUBLIC ACCESS

SCORE _____ /15   PASS ☐

7) DOG AND HANDLER CAN MANEUVER STAIRS OR ELEVATOR	TEAMWORK FOCUS APPROPRIATE FOR PUBLIC ACCESS

SCORE _____ /15   PASS ☐

8) TEAM HAS A SEAT AT A FOOD ESTABLISHMENT, DOG GOES UNDER SEAT/TABLE OR OTHERWISE POSITIONS ITSELF OUT OF THE WAY	TEAMWORK FOCUS APPROPRIATE FOR PUBLIC ACCESS

SCORE _____ /15   PASS ☐

9) DOG SHOWS APPROPRIATE RESPONSE WHEN FOOD IS DROPPED	TEAMWORK FOCUS APPROPRIATE FOR PUBLIC ACCESS

SCORE _____ /15   PASS ☐

10) DOG IGNORES PATRONS WHO ATTEMPT TO DISTRACT THEM	TEAMWORK FOCUS APPROPRIATE FOR PUBLIC ACCESS

SCORE _____ /15   PASS ☐

11) DOG REMAINS QUIET AND IN PLACE DURING MEAL	TEAMWORK FOCUS APPROPRIATE FOR PUBLIC ACCESS

SCORE _____ /15   PASS ☐

| 12) DOG REMAINS FOCUSED AND IN POSITION THROUGHOUT ESTABLISHMENT WITHOUT SNIFFING DISPLAYS OR OTHER PEOPLE | TEAMWORK
FOCUS
APPROPRIATE FOR PUBLIC ACCESS |

SCORE _____ /15   PASS ☐

| 13) DOG SHOWS APPROPRIATE RESPONSE TO VISUAL AND NOISE DISTRACTION | TEAMWORK
FOCUS
APPROPRIATE FOR PUBLIC ACCESS |

SCORE _____ /15   PASS ☐

| 14) HANDLER IS IN CONTROL WHEN EXITING THE BUILDING | TEAMWORK
FOCUS
APPROPRIATE FOR PUBLIC ACCESS |

SCORE _____ /15   PASS ☐

| 15) DOG IS CLEAN AND WELL-GROOMED | APPROPRIATE FOR PUBLIC ACCESS ☐ |

SCORE _____ /15   PASS ☐

| 16) SAFETY IS OBSERVED BY SECURING DOG IN A CANINE SEATBELT OR CRATE.IN THE VEHICLE | APPROPRIATE FOR PUBLIC ACCESS ☐ |

SCORE _____ /15   PASS ☐

| 17) HANDLER IS PREPARED FOR POTENTIAL ACCESS CHALLENGES | APPROPRIATE FOR PUBLIC ACCESS ☐ |

SCORE _____ /15   PASS ☐

| 18) HANDLER DEMONSTRATES PROPER USE OF GEAR AND/OR TRAINING AIDS | APPROPRIATE FOR PUBLIC ACCESS ☐ |

SCORE _____ /15   PASS ☐

| 19) OVERALL, DOG FOCUSES ON/RESPONDS TO HANDLER | APPROPRIATE FOR PUBLIC ACCESS ☐ |

SCORE _____ /15   PASS ☐

| 20) HANDLER IS PREPARED WITH SUPPLIES FOR DOG WASTE | APPROPRIATE FOR PUBLIC ACCESS ☐ |

SCORE _____ /15   PASS ☐

NOTES

FINAL SCORE

TEAMWORK _____ /100

FOCUS _____ /100

APPROPRIATE FOR
PUBLIC ACCESS _____ /100

☐ PASS   ☐ DID NOT PASS

EVALUATOR INFORMATION

NAME: _____

QUALIFICATIONS: _____

PHONE: _____

SIGNATURE: _____

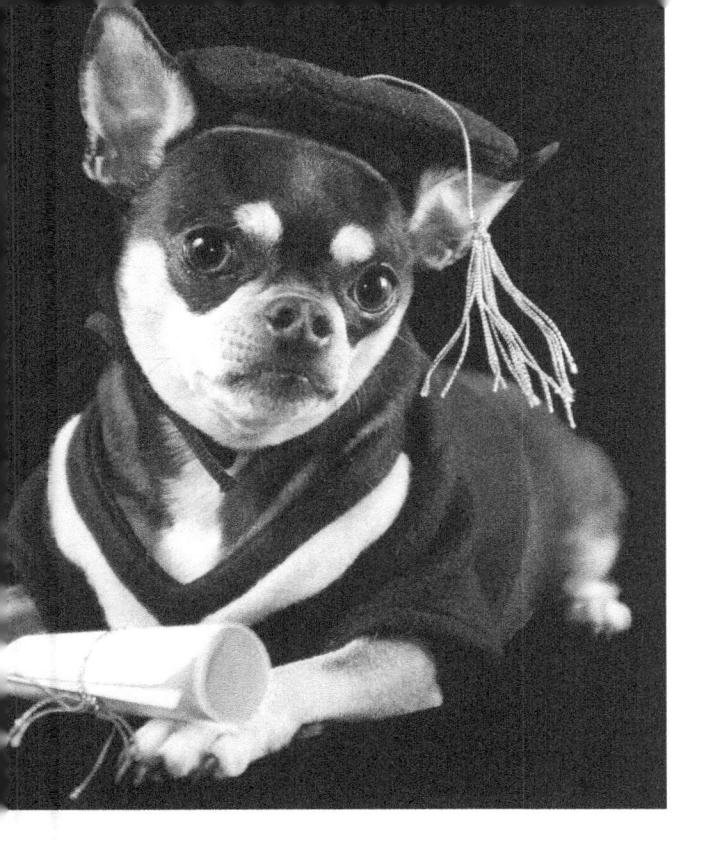

SCORING

1. EXCEPTIONAL

No mistakes, dog is comfortable, and focused on handler. Responds to cues immediately

2. GOOD

No mistakes, dog appears comfortable, Focused on handler most of the time, responds to all cues with no distraction

All portions must score 3 or above to pass the examination

3. ACCEPTABLE

Very few mistakes, dog appears comfortable, responds to cues with little distraction

4. NEEDS MORE TRAINING

Multiple mistakes, distracted/not focused on handler, mild stress signs, does not respond to cues

5. UNSUITABLE FOR PUBLIC ACCESS WORK

Extreme stress, Aggression, growling, fearfulness, noise sensitive

Congratulations! You have completed the last lesson in this book. If you have followed the program, you and your dog have learned many new skills and communication is better than ever between you.

Of course, training in not finished. No, training will continue throughout your dog's career as a service dog.

Generally speaking, a service dog should have a minimum of 120 hours of training with at least 30 hours of public access training before they will graduate from "in-training" status to full-fledged service dog.

Do not worry, I have plenty more for you! If you are raising a puppy, check out Volume III of this series. Volume VI is in the works now and will cover task training that builds on the foundation that you have learned in this workbook and in Volume V.

My readers are encouraged to reach out to me and tell me about their experiences in training.

If there are any struggles that I can help you work out I would love to hear from you. Specific challenges that you may encounter in training your dog while working with a condition that causes limitations can be really hard and I want to be able to help my readers overcome any challenge no matter the limitation.

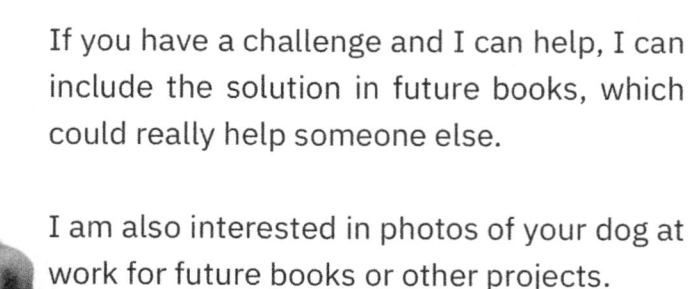

If you have a challenge and I can help, I can include the solution in future books, which could really help someone else.

I am also interested in photos of your dog at work for future books or other projects.

Be proud of yourself and your service dog team, you are doing it!

Good Luck!

ONE LAST THING...

If you enjoyed this book or found it useful I'd be very grateful if you'd post a short review on Amazon. Your support really does make a difference and I read all the reviews personally so I can get your feedback and make this book even better.

The next 2 books in this series are in the works as well, so keep your eyes peeled for them if you enjoyed the books in this series.

Thanks again for your support!

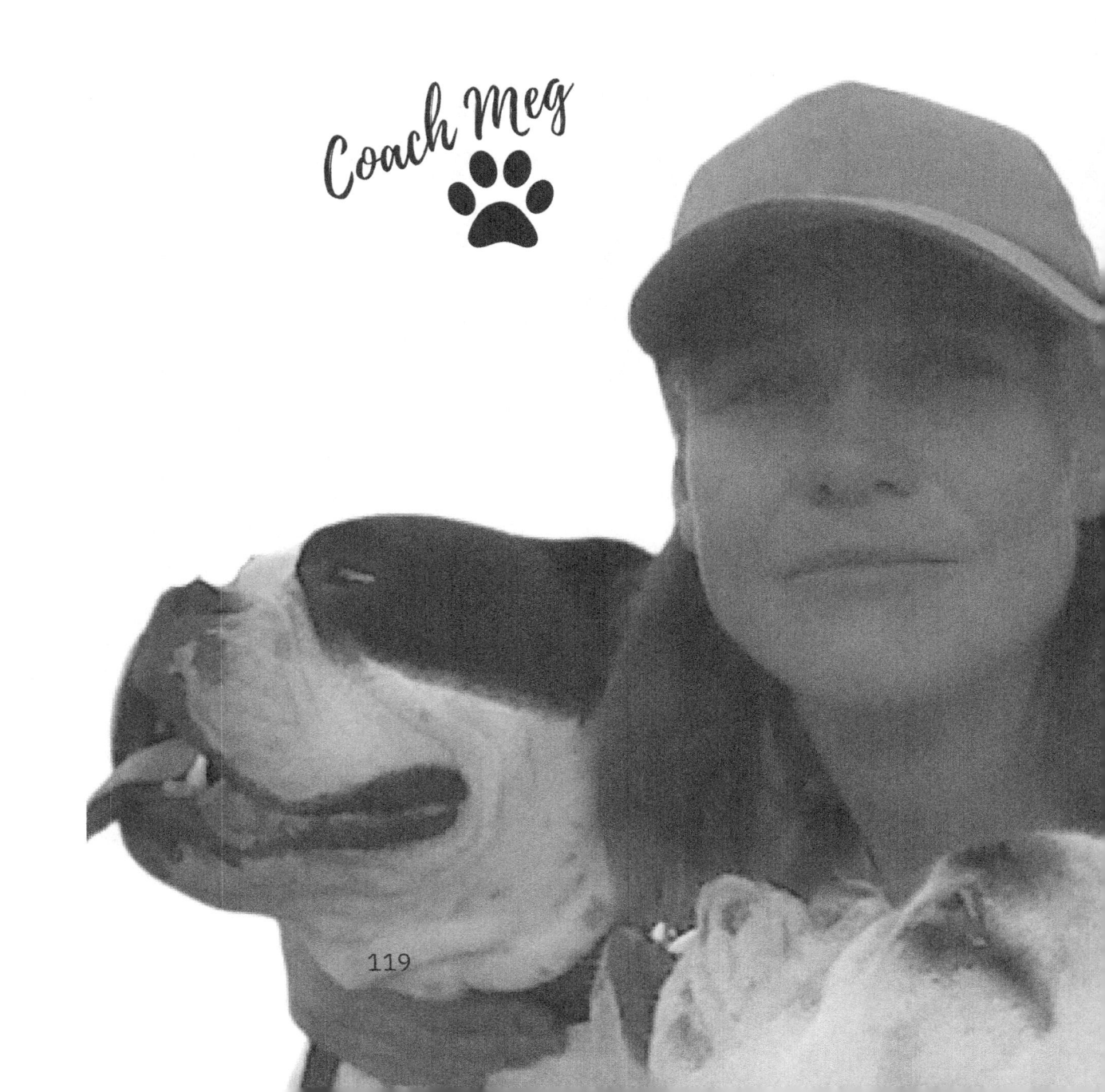

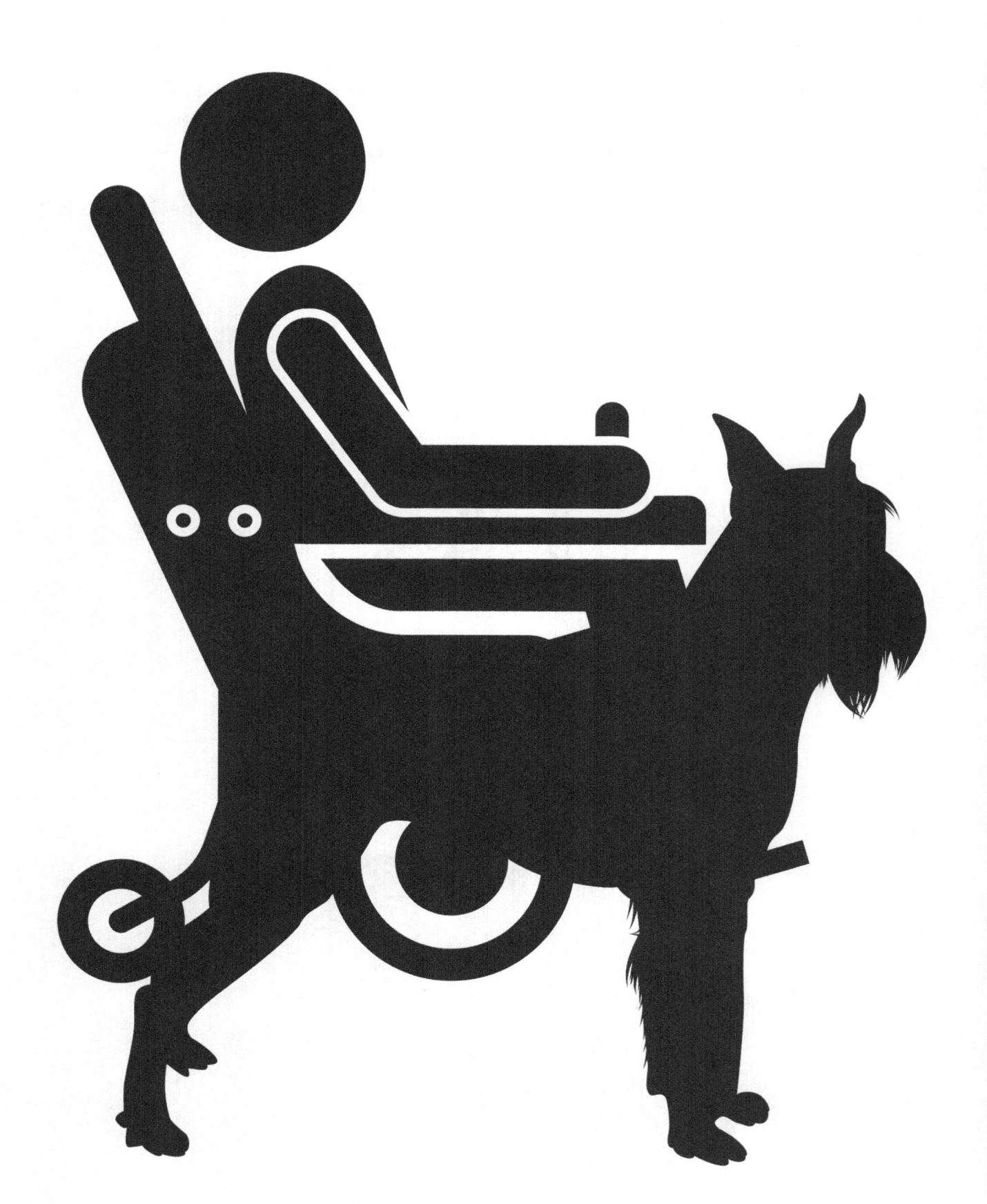

CHAPTER 13: WORKSHEETS

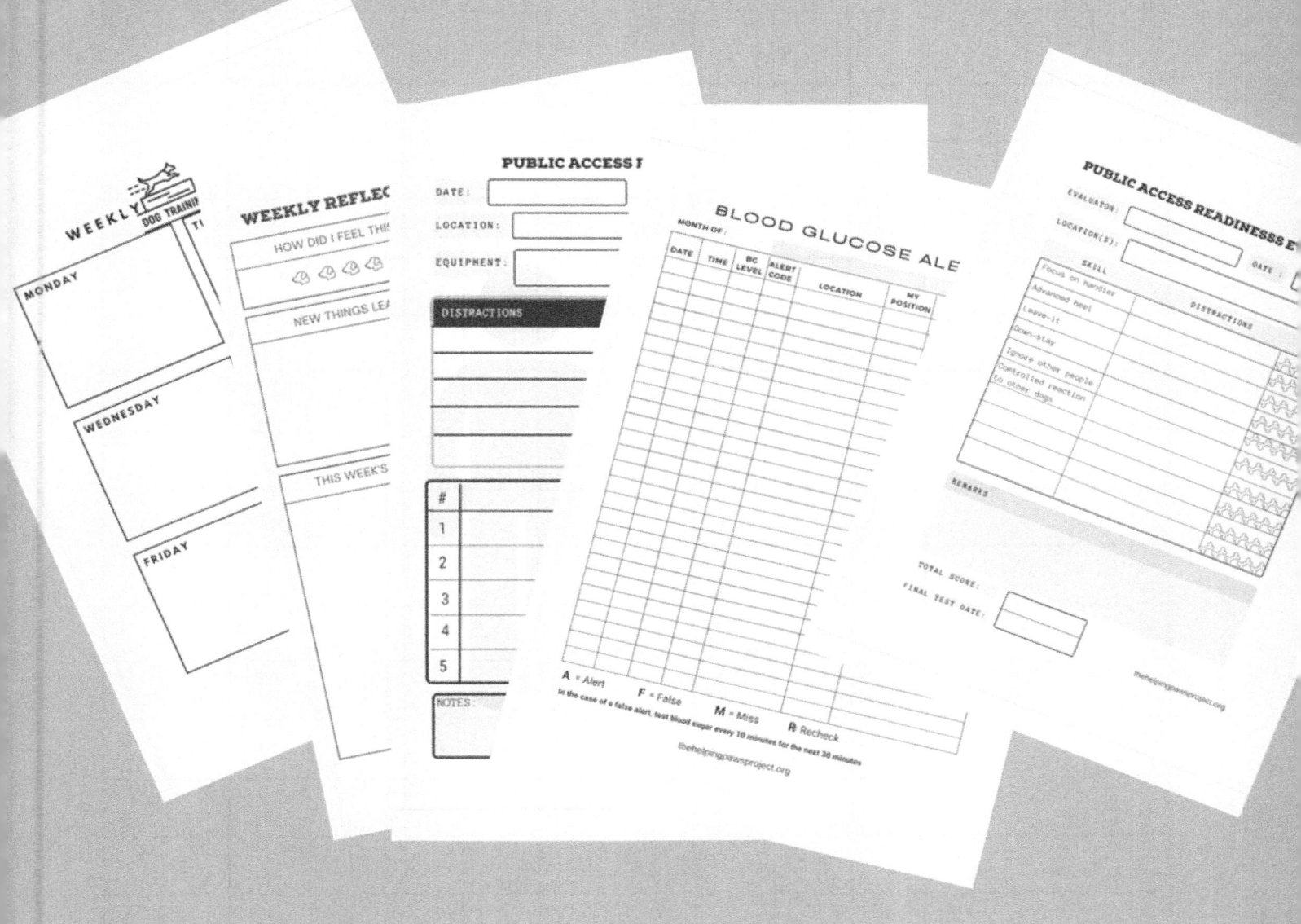

PUBLIC ACCESS HOURS

LOCATION	TIME LOGGED											TOTAL

PUBLIC ACCESS HOURS

LOCATION	TIME LOGGED										TOTAL

PUBLIC ACCESS HOURS

LOCATION				TIME LOGGED							TOTAL

PUBLIC ACCESS HOURS

LOCATION	TIME LOGGED									TOTAL

PUBLIC ACCESS PRACTICE JOURNAL

DATE: _____ ASSISTED BY: _____

LOCATION: _____

EQUIPMENT: _____

DISTRACTIONS

_____
_____
_____
_____

#	SKILL:	
1		☐ Needs Work
2		☐ Needs Work
3		☐ Needs Work
4		☐ Needs Work
5		☐ Needs Work

NOTES:

PUBLIC ACCESS PRACTICE JOURNAL

DATE: _____ **ASSISTED BY:** _____

LOCATION: _____

EQUIPMENT: _____

DISTRACTIONS

#	SKILL:	
1		☐ Needs Work
2		☐ Needs Work
3		☐ Needs Work
4		☐ Needs Work
5		☐ Needs Work

NOTES:

PUBLIC ACCESS PRACTICE JOURNAL

DATE: _____ **ASSISTED BY:** _____

LOCATION: _____

EQUIPMENT: _____

DISTRACTIONS

#	SKILL:	
1		☐ Needs Work
2		☐ Needs Work
3		☐ Needs Work
4		☐ Needs Work
5		☐ Needs Work

NOTES:

PUBLIC ACCESS PRACTICE JOURNAL

DATE: _____   ASSISTED BY: _____

LOCATION: _____

EQUIPMENT: _____

DISTRACTIONS

#	SKILL:	
1		☐ Needs Work
2		☐ Needs Work
3		☐ Needs Work
4		☐ Needs Work
5		☐ Needs Work

NOTES:

PUBLIC ACCESS PRACTICE JOURNAL

DATE: _____ ASSISTED BY: _____

LOCATION: _____

EQUIPMENT: _____

DISTRACTIONS

#	SKILL:	
1		☐ Needs Work
2		☐ Needs Work
3		☐ Needs Work
4		☐ Needs Work
5		☐ Needs Work

NOTES:

TASK TRAINING TRACKER

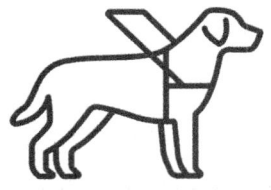

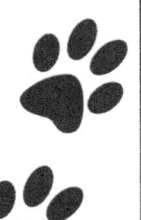

TASK	S	M	T	W	T	F	S
🐾							
🐾							
🐾							
🐾							
🐾							
🐾							
🐾							
🐾							
🐾							
🐾							

NOTES

TASK TRAINING TRACKER

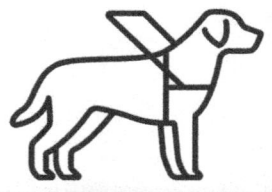

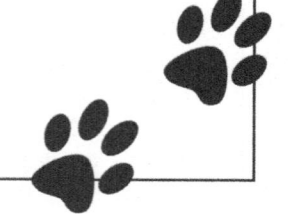

TASK	S	M	T	W	T	F	S
🐾							
🐾							
🐾							
🐾							
🐾							
🐾							
🐾							
🐾							
🐾							
🐾							

NOTES

TASK TRAINING TRACKER

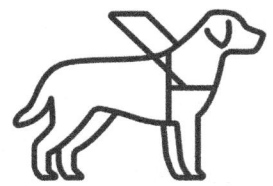

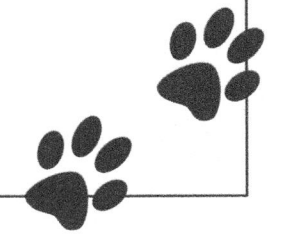

TASK	S	M	T	W	T	F	S
🐾							
🐾							
🐾							
🐾							
🐾							
🐾							
🐾							
🐾							
🐾							
🐾							

NOTES

TASK TRAINING TRACKER

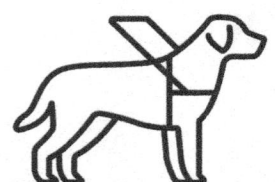

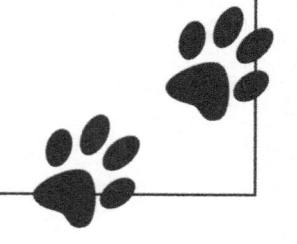

TASK	S	M	T	W	T	F	S
🐾							
🐾							
🐾							
🐾							
🐾							
🐾							
🐾							
🐾							
🐾							
🐾							

NOTES

PUBLIC ACCESS TRAINING OVERVIEW

Dog/Handler: _____ Date:: _____

Location: _____ Duration: _____

Atmosphere: _____

_____

Stress signals present? :   Yes   No

Behaviors/Tasks Practiced

_____
_____
_____
_____
_____
_____
_____

Challenges

Distractions

Overall Rating Today

Initial

PUBLIC ACCESS TRAINING OVERVIEW

Dog/Handler: _____ Date:: _____

Location: _____ Duration: _____

Atmosphere: _____

_____

Stress signals present? : Yes   No

Behaviors/Tasks Practiced

Challenges	Distractions

Overall Rating Today
🦴 🦴 🦴 🦴 🦴 🦴 🦴 🦴 🦴 🦴

Initial

136

PUBLIC ACCESS TRAINING OVERVIEW

Dog/Handler: _____ Date:: _____

Location: _____ Duration: _____

Atmosphere: _____

_____

Stress signals present? :   Yes   No

Behaviors/Tasks Practiced

Challenges

Distractions

Overall Rating Today

Initial

PUBLIC ACCESS TRAINING OVERVIEW

Dog/Handler: _____   Date:: _____

Location: _____   Duration: _____

Atmosphere: _____

_____

Stress signals present? :   Yes   No

Behaviors/Tasks Practiced

Challenges

Distractions

Overall Rating Today

Initial

Training Step Planning Tool

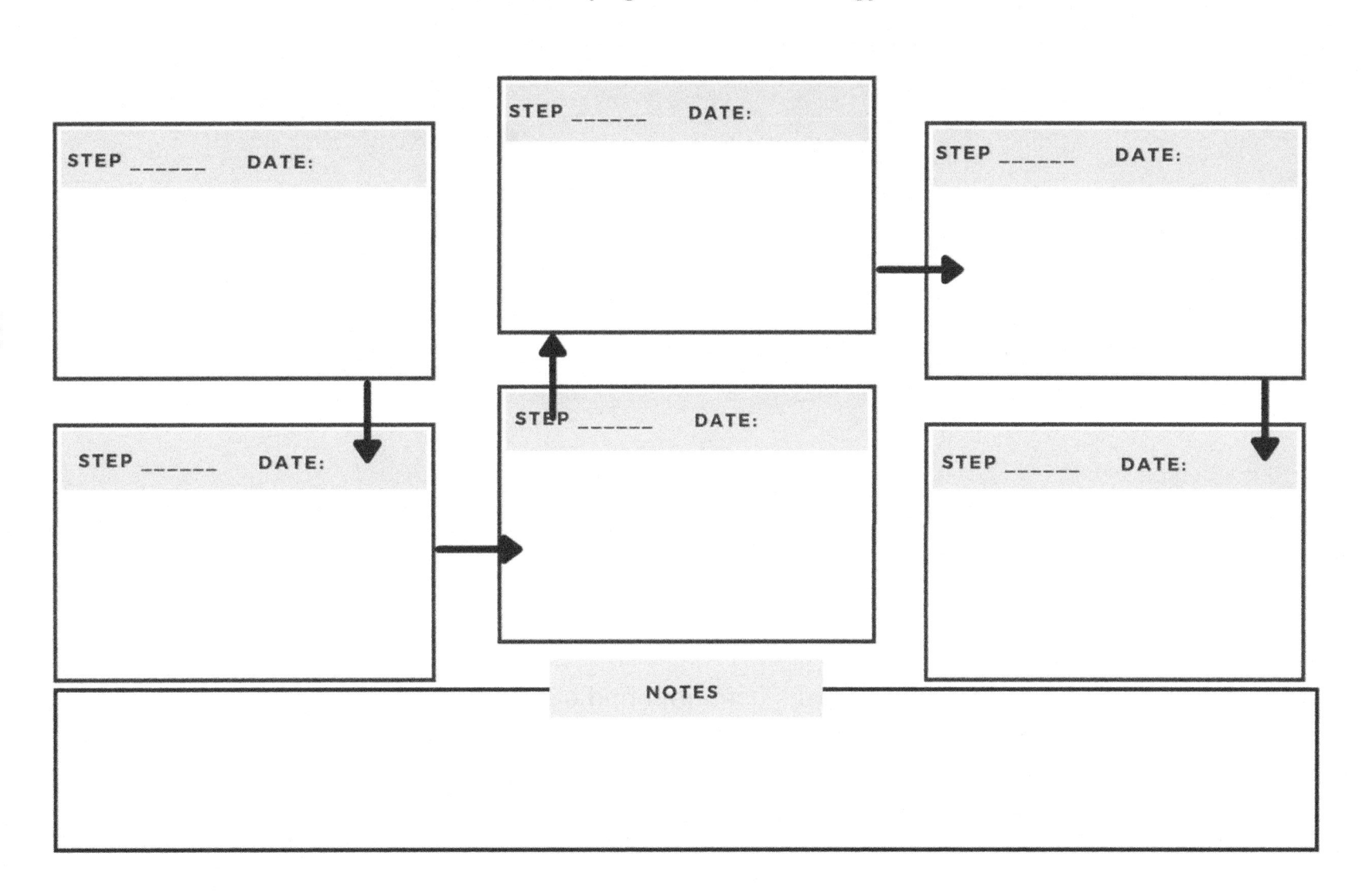

Action Plan

DATE:

Break one strategy down into steps, these steps become your daily tasks.
Use one page for each strategy.

STEP ____ DATE: ____

STEP ____ DATE: ____

STEP ____ DATE: ____

STEP ____ DATE: ____

STEP ____ DATE: ____

STEP ____ DATE: ____

NOTES

Training Step Planning Tool

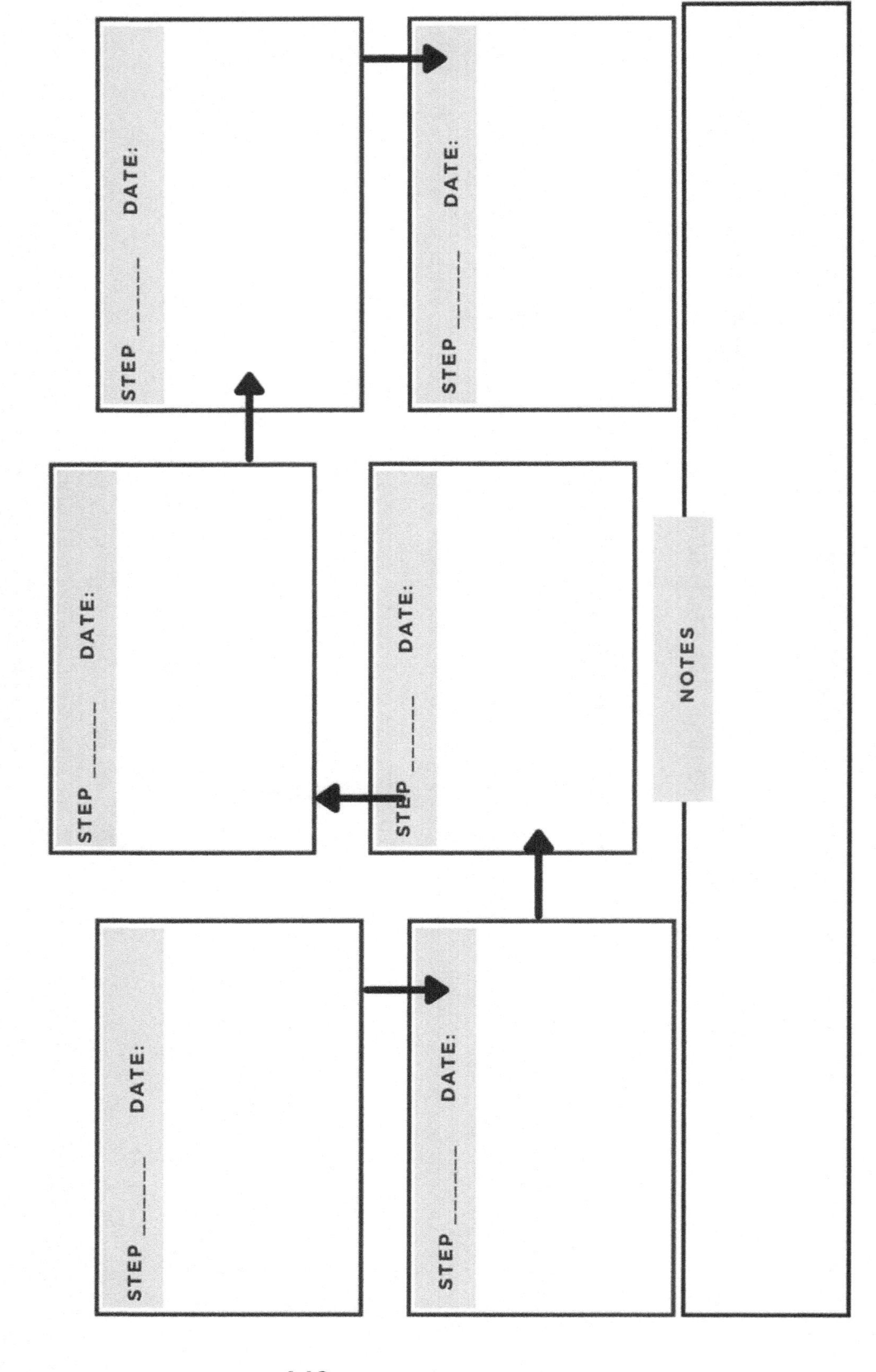

Action Plan

DATE:

Break one strategy down into steps, these steps become your daily tasks. Use one page for each strategy.

STEP _____ DATE: ____

STEP _____ DATE: ____

STEP _____ DATE: ____

STEP _____ DATE: ____

STEP _____ DATE: ____

STEP _____ DATE: ____

NOTES

Training Step Planning Tool

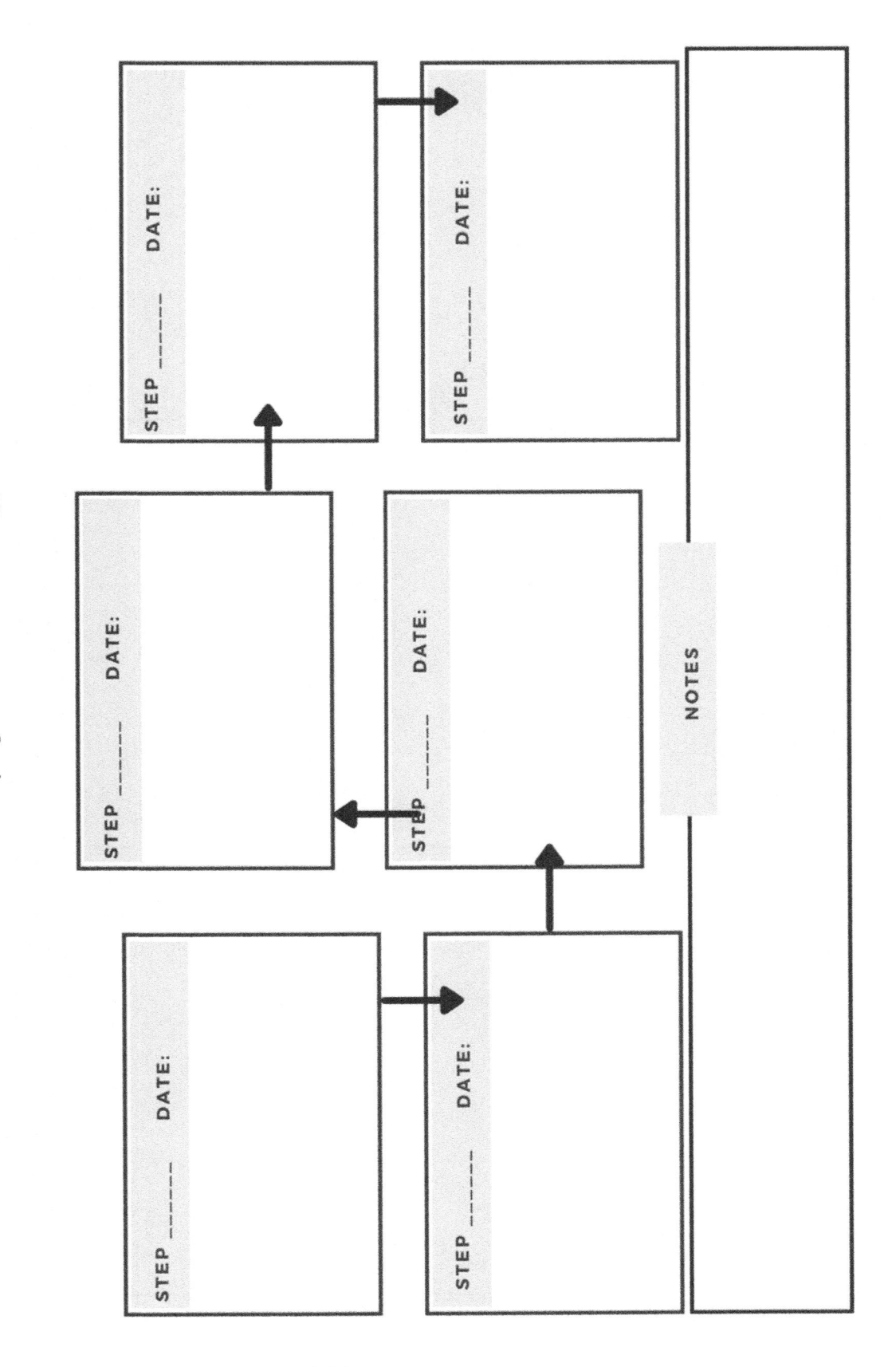

Action Plan

DATE:

Break one strategy down into steps, these steps become your daily tasks. Use one page for each strategy.

STEP ____ DATE: ____	STEP ____ DATE: ____

STEP ____ DATE: ____	STEP ____ DATE: ____

STEP ____ DATE: ____	STEP ____ DATE: ____

NOTES

Training Step Planning Tool

Action Plan

DATE:

Break one strategy down into steps, these steps become your daily tasks. Use one page for each strategy.

STEP _____ DATE: ____

STEP _____ DATE: ____

STEP _____ DATE: ____

STEP _____ DATE: ____

STEP _____ DATE: ____

STEP _____ DATE: ____

NOTES

SAMPLE LETTER FOR PERMISSION TO TRAIN IN AN ESTABLISHMENT

(Date)

Manager/Owner's Name
Name of Establishment
Address of Establishment

Your name
(Dog's Name) Service Dog in Training
Contact information

Dear (name of person in charge or establishment name),

My name is (your name) and I work with a service dog in training, (dog's name), who is being trained to assist me with a disability. (Dog's name) is learning to assist me by performing tasks such as: (optional: list any tasks).

After approximately (state an estimated number of hours using your training logs) hours of intensive training, I feel that (dog's name) is ready to begin public access training in order to complete training and graduate to full service dog status.

While federal law protects my right to use a service dog in places open to the public, it does not specifically mention service dogs in training.

For this reason, and because (establishment) is a place I come to regularly, I am requesting permission to have (Dog's name) accompany me and complete the public access portion of his/her training.

This would be extremely helpful for us to develop the skills necessary for recognition as a full-fledged service dog team.

(The following portion is optional but can be helpful if the person is reluctant and you really need them to agree)

Please keep in mind; my SDiT has undergone a great deal of training to ensure that he/she is ready to perform professionally in public places.

I have drawn up an agreement if you would feel more comfortable, that attests to acceptable behavior on my team's part.

We are willing to meet with you in person so you to observe (dog's name) level of training if it would be helpful in making a favorable decision.

Thank you for your time and consideration in this matter.

(Make sure that you give a specific call-to-action and tell the recipient what you need)

I will contact you on (date) for your decision or you can contact me sooner if you prefer.

Sincerely
(Your signature)

(Printed name)

OPTIONAL AGREEMENT ATTESTING TO BEHAVIOR OF A SERVICE DOG IN TRAINING
FOR RELUCTANT ESTABLISHMENTS

I,_____, attest to the level of training my service dog-in-training *(SDiT)* _____,has achieved in preparation for public access work.

In receiving permission to visit this establishment with the said *SDiT* for training purposes, I certify the following to be true to the best of my knowledge.

My Service Dog in Training is:

- [ ] Non-aggressive
- [ ] Housebroken
- [ ] Current on license and vaccinations as required by the city and is in good health
- [ ] Clean and well-groomed
- [ ] Under my control at all times
- [ ] Expected to focus on me and not seek attention from other people
- [ ] Leashed/tethered at all times unless a task requires the leash to be removed

I understand I am liable for damages should they ever occur.

I agree that if at any time my service dog's behavior was to cause a disruption (barking, harassing other people, eliminating indoors) and I am not able to regain control of my dog, I will leave the establishment and continue training prior to attempting public access again.

By signing this document, you agree to extend permission to this service dog team for purposes of service dog training.

Representative Name (Print): _____

Name of Establishment: _____

Signature: _____ Date: _____

Service Dog Handler's Name (Print): _____

Signature: _____ Date: _____

ADA Information Line
Phone: 800-514-0301 (voice) or 800-514-0383 (TTY)
at
US Department of Justice
950 Pennsylvania Avenue, NW
Civil Rights Division
Disability Rights Section – NYA
Washington, D.C. 20530

Disability Rights Education & Defense Fund (DREDF)
3075 Adeline Street, Suite 210
Berkeley, CA 94703
Phone: 510-644-2555 (voice) or 510-841-8645 (fax/TTY)
info@dref.org

US Access Board
(Architectural and Transportation Barriers Compliance Board)
1331 F Street NW, Suite 1000
Washington, DC 2004-1111
Phone: 1-800- 872-2253 (voice) or 1-800-993-2822 (TTY)

ADA Service Animal Resource Hub
https://adata.org/service-animal-resource-hub

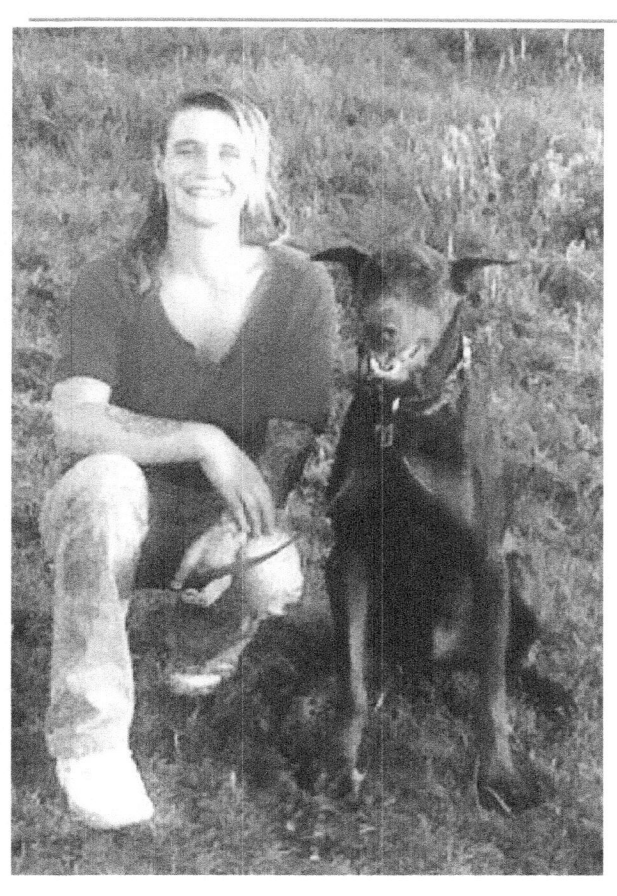

ABOUT THE AUTHOR

Megan Brooks is a professional dog trainer who has worked with dogs for as long as she can remember. She has specialized in service dog training since 2008.

Megan worked as a Certified Veterinary Technician in the Denver area until she was permanently injured in a motor vehicle accident in 2003.

This is when Megan trained her own dog for mobility assistance and started The Helping Paws Project to help other people with disabilities train their own pets for service dog work.

in 2008, Megan earned her CDT (Certified Dog Trainer) through the International Association of Canine Professionals (IACP)and has been an AKC Canine Good Citizen Evaluator since 2008 as well.

Megan currently resides in Northern New Mexico where she continues to run the Helping Paws Project & Bulldogs for Soldiers. She also volunteers at the Reuse Center, a recycling/donation facility.
She shares life with 3 Bulldogs, 2 horses, a cat, and an African Grey Parrot.

Other Books by Megan Brooks

TRAINING YOUR OWN SERVICE DOG THE COMPLETE GUIDE SERIES

- • Volume I Training your Service Dog The Complete Guide Series
- • Volume II Training your Service Dog The Complete Guide Series: Basic Obedience Skills Workbook
- • Volume III Training your Service Dog The Complete Guide Series: Raising your Service Dog Puppy
- • Volume IV Training your Service Dog The Complete Guide Series: Public Access Skills Workbook
- • Volume V Training your Service Dog The Complete Guide Series: Foundations (Coming Soon)
- Volume VI Training your Service Dog The Complete Guide Series: Task Training (Coming Soon)

What Your Pet Wants You to Know the Truth About Commercial Pet Food: Pet Food Dangers Exposed

No Dogs Allowed: The Business Owners Guide to ADA Service Dog Law

HOW TO WIN YOUR SOCIAL SECURITY CLAIM FAST! SERIES

- • Volume I How to Win Your Social Security Claim FAST! Secrets to a Successful SSDI Claim
- • Volume II How to Win Your Social Security Claim FAST! Workbook
- • Volume III How to Win Your Social Security Claim FAST! Medical Treatment Journal

RESOURCES

- AKC Temperament Test – American Kennel Club
https://www.akc.org/akctemptest/

- AKC Trick Dog – American Kennel Club
https://www.akc.org/sports/trick-dog/

- AKC Therapy Dog – American Kennel Club
https://www.akc.org/sports/title-recognition-program/therapy-dog-program/

About Community Canine – American Kennel Club
https://www.akc.org/products-services/training-programs/canine-good-citizen/akc-community-canine/

International Association of Assistance Dog Partners
https://iaadp.org/

Psychiatric Service Dog Partners (tons of resources for all types of service dog teams)
https://www.psychdogpartners.org/resources/public-access/public-access-test
https://www.psychdogpartners.org/resources/public-access/manners-evaluation

Anything Pawsable (great source of resources)
https://anythingpawsable.com/training

OTHER BOOKS IN THE
TRAINING YOUR OWN SERVICE DOG (THE COMPLETE GUIDE) SERIES

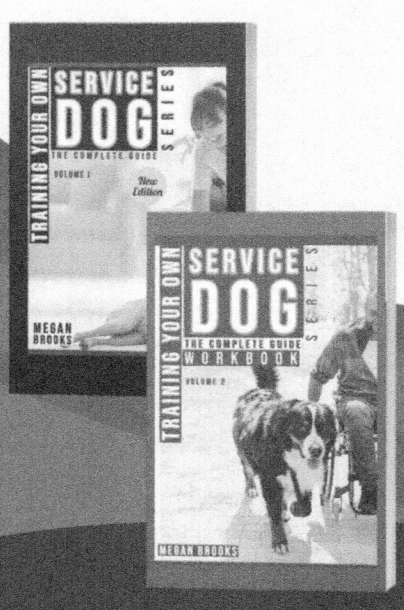

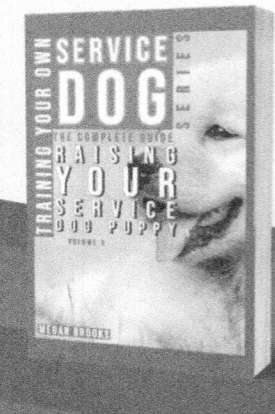

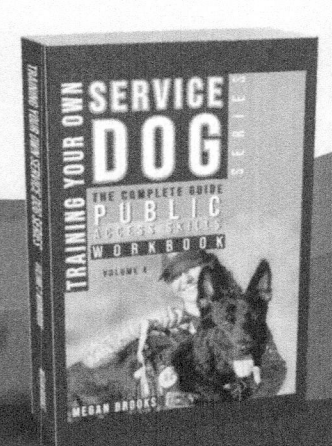

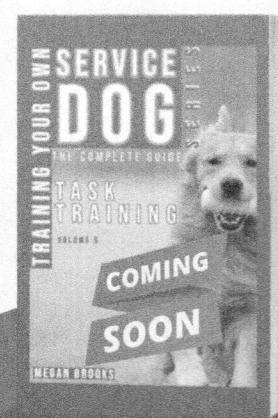

Written by Professional Service Dog Trainer and Certified Life Coach, Megan Brooks.

Coach Meg "The Dog Trainer" has trained more than 100 service dog teams and helped dozens of people like you train their own dog to help them.

Contact Us

https://thehelpingpawsproject.org
helpingpawsservicedogs@gmail.com

What's In The Series?

- ✓ Complete ADA service dog law
- ✓ Understanding your rights and responsibilities
- ✓ Training effectively using my MEGA LEARN System
- ✓ Public access ready in 2 weeks
- ✓ 100+ tasks you can train (coming soon)
- ✓ And much much more!

FOR SALE ON AMAZON

READY TO WIN YOUR SOCIAL SECURITY DISABILITY CLAIM THE FIRST TIME WITHOUT PAYING AN ATTORNEY?

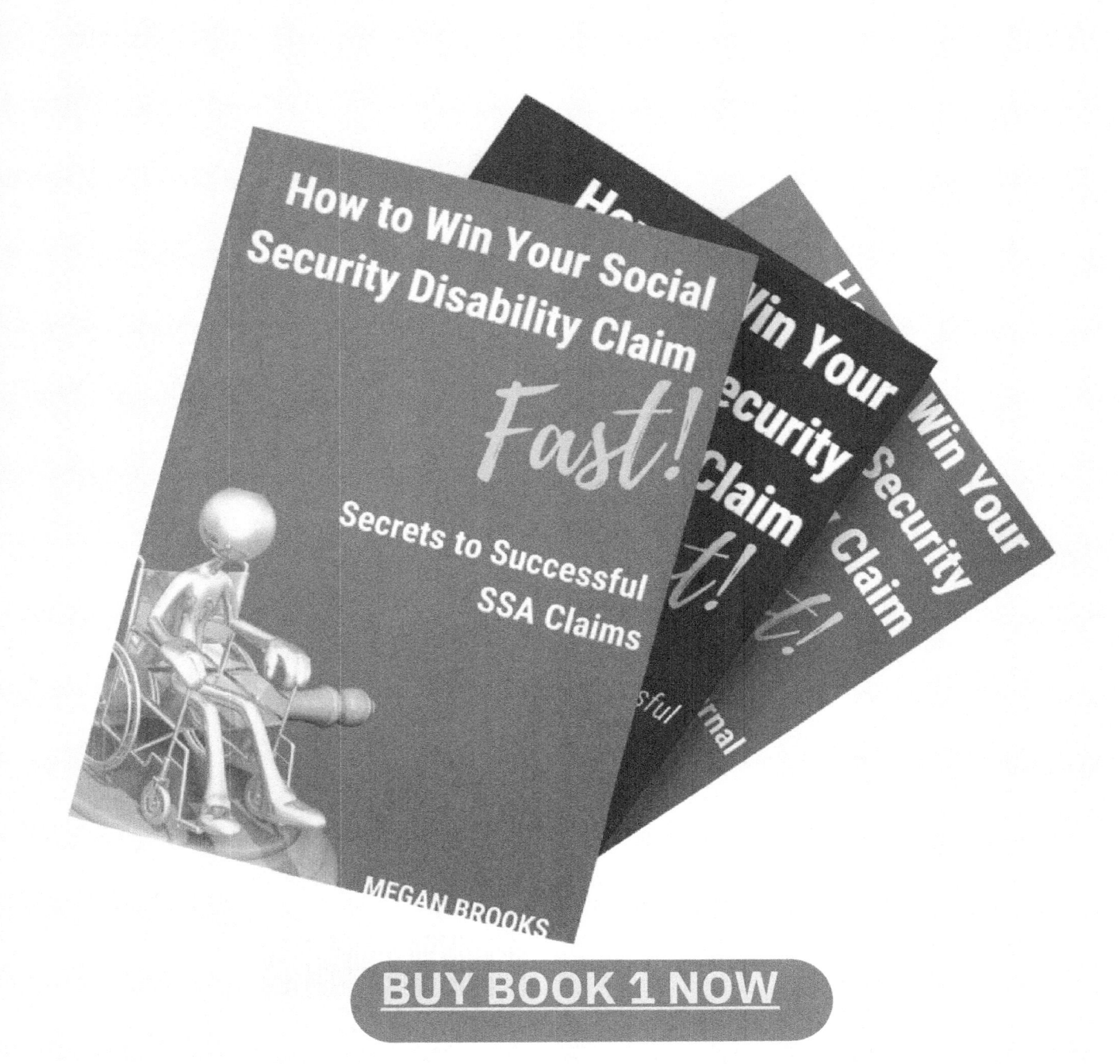

BUY BOOK 1 NOW

FOR SALE ON AMAZON.COM

Made in the USA
Monee, IL
05 June 2023